MAJOR PROBLEMS IN INTERNAL MEDICINE

Published

Cline: Cancer Chemotherapy (third edition by Cline and Haskell now available separately)
Shearn: Sjögren's Syndrome
Cogan: Ophthalmic Manifestations of Systemic Vascular Disease
Williams: Rheumatoid Arthritis as a Systemic Disease
Cluff, Caranasos and Stewart: Clinical Problems with Drugs
Fries and Holman: Systemic Lupus Erythematosus
Kass: Pernicious Anemia
Braude: Antimicrobial Drug Therapy
Bray: The Obese Patient
Zieve and Levin: Bleeding Disorders
Gorlin: Coronary Artery Disease
Bunn, Forget and Ranney: Hemoglobinopathies
Sleisenger and Brandborg: Malabsorption
Beeson and Bass: The Eosinophil
Krugman and Gocke: Viral Hepatitis
Hurwitz, Duranceau, and Haddad: Disorders of Esophageal Motility
Galambos: Cirrhosis
Nelson: The Adrenal Cortex: Physiological Function and Disease
Raskin and Appenzeller: Headache
Brooks: Disorders of the Exocrine Pancreas
Cupps and Fauci: The Vasculitides
Lieber: Medical Disorders of Alcoholism—Pathogenesis and Treatment

MAJOR PROBLEMS IN INTERNAL MEDICINE

In Preparation

Potts: Disorders of Calcium Metabolism
James and Williams: Sarcoidosis
Atkins and Bodel: Fever
Goldberg: The Scientific Basis and Practical Use of Diuretics
Kilbourne: Influenza
Cohen: Amyloidosis
Durie: Multiple Myeloma
Weinstein: Infective Endocarditis
Sasahara: Pulmonary Embolism
Swartz: Meningitis
Sparling: Venereal Diseases
McLees: Critical Care
Engel: Psychosocial Problems in Medical Practice
Utz: Systemic Mycotic Infections
Walser and Mitch: Conservative Management of Renal Failure
Chatterjee: Medical Problems in the Coronary Care Unit

I. HERBERT SCHEINBERG, M.D.

Professor of Medicine and Head, Division of Genetic Medicine,
Albert Einstein College of Medicine;
Attending Physician, Bronx Municipal Hospital Center, Bronx, New York

IRMIN STERNLIEB, M.D.

Professor of Medicine and Associate Director, Liver Research Center,
Albert Einstein College of Medicine;
Attending Physician, Bronx Municipal Hospital Center, Bronx, New York

WILSON'S DISEASE

VOLUME

XXIII

IN THE SERIES

MAJOR PROBLEMS IN INTERNAL MEDICINE

Lloyd H. Smith, Jr., M.D., *Editor*

1984

W. B. SAUNDERS COMPANY

PHILADELPHIA • LONDON • TORONTO • MEXICO CITY • RIO DE JANEIRO • SYDNEY • TOKYO

W. B. Saunders Company: West Washington Square
Philadelphia, PA 19105

1 St. Anne's Road
Eastbourne, East Sussex BN21 3UN, England

1 Goldthorne Avenue
Toronto, Ontario M8Z 5T9, Canada

Apartado 26370—Cedro 512
Mexico 4, D.F., Mexico

Rua Coronel Cabrita, 8
Sao Cristovao Caixa Postal 21176
Rio de Janeiro, Brazil

9 Waltham Street
Artarmon, N.S.W. 2064, Australia

Ichibancho, Central Bldg., 22-1 Ichibancho
Chiyoda-Ku, Tokyo 102, Japan

Library of Congress Cataloging in Publication Data

Scheinberg, I. Herbert.

Wilson's disease.

Major problems in internal medicine ; v. 23)
1. Hepatolenticular degeneration—Addresses, essays, lectures. I. Sternlieb, Irmin. II. Title. III. Series. [DNLM: 1. Hepatolenticular degeneration.

W1 MA492T v.23 / WI740 S319w]

RC394.H4S34 1984 616.3′62 83-14271

ISBN 0-7216-7953-6

Wilson's Disease ISBN 7216-7953-6

Last digit is the print number: 9 8 7 6 5 4 3 2 1

Dedicated

to

John M. Walshe

FOREWORD

Metabolic diseases are usually diseases of too little or too much. The body's economy of virtually all of its constituents is relatively precisely tuned, fat in adipose tissues being one of the few exceptions. Here, excess calories are packaged in innumerable cellular containers against presumed future needs. For most metabolic products, however, and for most dietary constituents, there must be a careful accounting of that in use and that in inventory. The homeostasis is generally less precise than that which maintains the internal milieu, but nevertheless it must be there.

These principles hold true for the inorganic cations that play such diverse roles in physiology, biochemistry, and structural integrity. These include sodium, potassium, calcium, magnesium, iron, copper, zinc, manganese, molybdenum, selenium, chromium, silicon, nickel, tin and vanadium. For those cations that are found in free solution in extracellular or intracellular fluid, there are beautifully balanced mechanisms of absorption and particularly of modulated excretion. These mechanisms often use hormones in their efferent pathways—for example, aldosterone, 1,25-dihydroxycholecalciferol and parathormone. Those metals that are primarily intracellular and serve as prosthetic elements for specific enzymes are often protein bound in extracellular fluid. The control of the body's stores of these cations is both more obscure and more subject to variation. No specific hormones have been detected, although they may possibly be there. How does the gut mucosa, for example, receive the signal that iron stores are enhanced or depleted or that erythropoiesis has been turned on or suppressed?

Eventually, we shall probably be able to develop a full panel of syndromes representing diseases of too little and too much of the body stores of these cations. There may well be subsets representing the time over which these aberrations have developed—acute versus chronic deficiency or excess. This information is now available for copper. No acute deficiency of copper has been recognized in man, but rarely chronic deficiency may be found, especially in infants. The abnormalities are mostly hematologic with anemia, leukopenia and maturation arrest. The abnormalities in copper metabolism found in Menkes' (steely-hair) disease, once thought to be due to a selective defect in copper absorption and therefore pure copper deficiency, are now known to be more complex. Disturbances in copper uptake and utilization in cultured cells (fibroblasts, lymphocytes, amniotic cells) can be demonstrated. Parenteral therapy with copper is not effective. Acute copper poisoning may occur during renal dialysis with equipment containing copper tubing, after intentional or accidental ingestion of copper salts, or after the absorption of copper sulfate through the skin during the treatment of burns. This may result in hemolytic anemia, centrilobular liver necrosis, rhabdomyolysis, nausea, vomiting, diarrhea, pancreatitis and gastrointestinal bleeding.

Most interest in copper metabolism in humans, however, has revolved around the rare but interesting genetic disorder termed Wilson's disease. Described more than 70 years ago (1912) by Samuel Alexander Kinnier Wilson as "progressive lenticular degeneration," Wilson's disease was found only one year later to be associated with increased copper in the liver. It was only in 1948, however, that excessive urinary excretion of copper was demonstrated in a typically serendipitous manner: the patient with Wilson's disease was being used as a control in a study designed to test for copper deficiency in multiple sclerosis! Following from this came the important observation that Wilson's disease represents chronic copper poisoning that can be prevented or reversed using chelating agents, especially D-penicillamine. The associated deficiency of ceruloplasmin was soon discovered by one of the authors of this monograph, I. Herbert Scheinberg, with David Gitlin, and in independent work by Alexander Bearn and Henry Kunkel (1952). Over the past 30 years, our understanding of the pathogenesis and clinical manifestations of Wilson's disease has been remarkably advanced, but the basic molecular defect that links the defective synthesis of ceruloplasmin and the defective biliary excretion of copper has not yet been elucidated.

In this monograph, Dr. Scheinberg and Dr. Sternlieb have presented a superb summary of current knowledge concerning Wilson's disease, based in considerable measure on their own research contributions and remarkable clinical experience with the disease. Although rare, Wilson's disease is of great importance in that effective treatment is available. The disease may present with the insidious onset of liver disease, of neurologic manifestations, of psychiatric disturbances, or of acute hemolytic anemia. It must therefore be frequently considered, although it is infrequently found. This treatise distills the scholarship of three decades of work by the authors. As such it is an admirable addition to our series of monographs on *Major Problems in Internal Medicine.*

LLOYD H. SMITH, JR., M.D.

Professor and Chairman,
Department of Medicine,
University of California, San Francisco

ACKNOWLEDGMENTS

In our study of Wilson's disease, in the care of our patients, and in the preparation of this monograph we have been skillfully and generously aided by our colleagues, including Philip Aisen, Maurice Eisenstadt, David Gitlin, Sidney Goldfischer, Phyllis S. Grushoff, Shalom Hirschman, Edith Korotkin, Jay Shapiro, Richard J. Stockert, Cornelius van den Hamer and Julie Windsor. Our debt to Anatol G. Morell—from whose wisdom, intuition, and scientific expertise we have drawn continually for thirty years—is beyond words.

Primarily because of the work of John Walshe, we have been fortunate in working on a disease that we have been able to treat effectively in the majority of our patients. Almost without exception, they have been willing (if not always eager) to undergo hospitalizations, biopsies, bloodletting, photographic sessions and a variety of clinical evaluations, despite their knowledge that these studies were unlikely to enable us to do more for them therapeutically. Each is referred to specifically by a letter-number code whenever we describe data derived from one of them. Whatever unique value this book may have is largely due to their participation in these studies, and we are very grateful to them. Jack Levin has not only allowed us to study him repeatedly, but has been tireless in contributing and raising financial support for The Foundation for the Study of Wilson's Disease.

Whenever necessary for their study, patients have been hospitalized in the General Clinical Research Center of the Albert Einstein College of Medicine–Bronx Municipal Hospital Center, whose Director, Quentin B. Deming, and staff have made it possible to carry out investigations accurately with concern for the comfort of the patients.

William F. Regan, Jr., generously provided the photographs he took, through a slit-lamp, of the Kayser-Fleischer rings of patient M15 (Color Plate 1, Figure 3).

The preparation of the electron micrographs was carried out, in large part, by Nelson Quintana. Photographs of all figures were made by George Dominguez.

Chapter 1 has been critically read by Christopher Lehmann-Haupt; Chapter 3, by Anatol Morell; Chapter 5, by Hans Popper; Chapter 6, by Dikran S. Horoupian; Chapter 9, by Charles Brenner and Morton F. Reiser; and Chapter 11, by Milford Fulop. Denis R. Giblin wrote a preliminary draft of Chapter 8, much of which we incorporated in its final version, which he also read critically.

Our investigations have been supported, in part, by grants from the National Institutes of Health (AM-1059, AM-17702, 5M01 RR-50, HD-00674 and CA-06576); The Commonwealth Fund; Merck, Sharp and Dohme; The Foundation for the Study of Wilson's Disease, Inc.; the Philip and Lynn Straus Foundation; and the Beth Paula Arenofsky, Yvonne Rogers, and Robert Schuldiner Memorial Funds.

I. HERBERT SCHEINBERG
IRMIN STERNLIEB

CONTENTS

WILSON'S DISEASE

PLATE 1

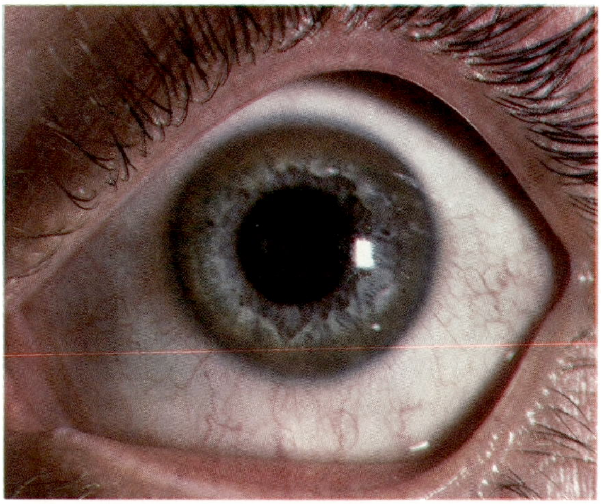

Figure 1. Kayser-Fleischer ring, at the periphery of the cornea, is a complete golden-brown circle that is more pronounced in the upper and lower quadrants. Patient T8.

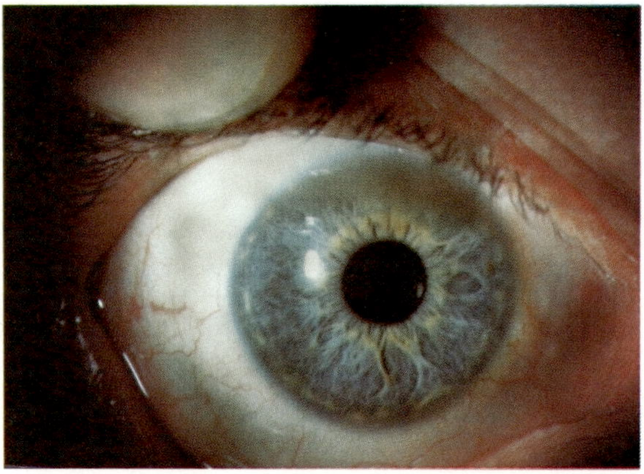

Figure 2. Fading Kayser-Fleischer rings appear as a broad crescent occupying about one half of the corneal radius in the superior quadrant, about one sixth of the corneal radius in somewhat more than the inferior quadrant, with no evidence of the ring laterally or medially. The patient, F10, is a 33-year-old man who has been treated with penicillamine since the diagnosis of Wilson's disease was made 16 years ago, at which time his rings were completely circumferential.

PLATE 2

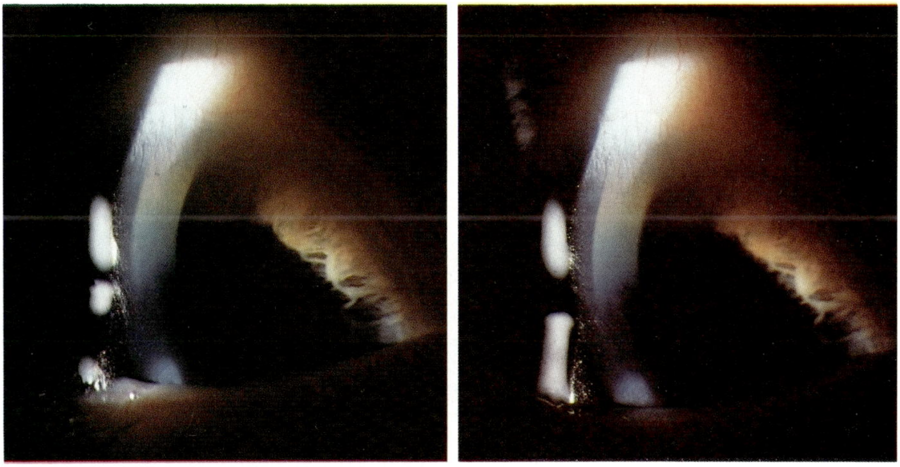

Figure 3. Stereoscopic photograph of a Kayser-Fleischer ring illuminated by a slit-lamp. The reader's eyes should be as close to the page as his nearpoint permits, and he should allow his eyes to diverge so that both images fuse. Patient M15. The hazy-gray surface of the curved parallelopiped is reflected from the anterior corneal surface; the golden surface, which fades toward the corneal center, is reflected from the Kayser-Fleischer ring in Descemet's membrane. Patient M15.

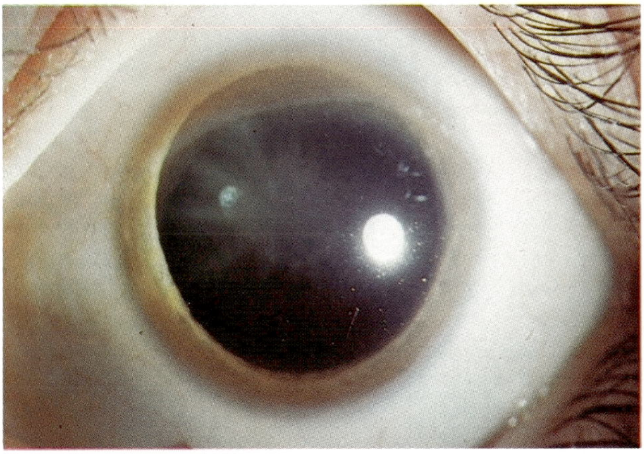

Figure 4. Sunflower cataract. Patient G10.

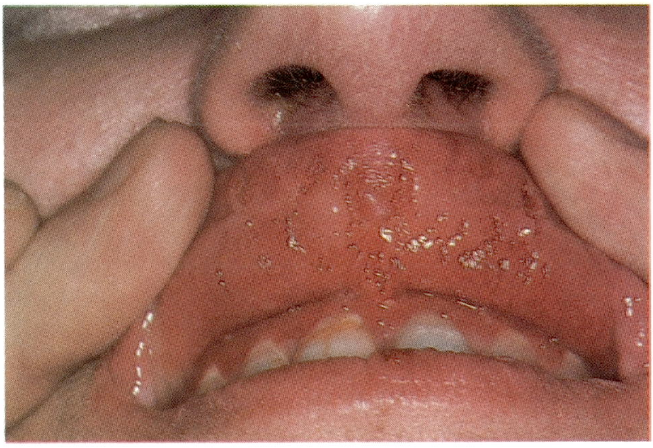

Figure 5. Vesiculobullous and erosive lesions characteristic of pemphigus involving the labial mucosa and gingiva. These lesions were of four years' duration in a 24-year-old woman, S19, treated with D-penicillamine for seven years. They disappeared after discontinuance of D-penicillamine and institution of Trien. (Courtesy Dr. Ellen Eisenberg.)

INTRODUCTION

This monograph is intended to be a critical summary of our knowledge of Wilson's disease. It is based primarily on the records of the authors' 30 years of experience in investigating, diagnosing and treating patients with Wilson's disease, as well as on the literature. In addition to histologic, ultrastructural, biochemical and genetic studies, we have directly cared for about 200 patients—some for more than 25 years—and have performed diagnostic and consultative services for perhaps another 300 patients.

We originally planned to title this volume "Wilson's Disease and Human Copper Metabolism," but during the preparation of the manuscript we recognized that these were in reality subjects for two different monographs. The only aspect of copper metabolism that is pathologically affected in Wilson's disease is the genetically transmitted mechanism that normally maintains equality between the amount of dietary copper absorbed and excreted. Wilson's disease is not in any other sense a significant disorder of copper metabolism—it is chronic copper toxicosis of man.

Nevertheless, brief reference to a few facts of the physiology and pathology of copper may be a useful background. Without it the reader might conclude that the most important distinction between Wilson's disease and other chronic heavy metal toxicoses, such as those of lead and mercury, is merely that Wilson's disease is caused by copper. In fact, the critical difference lies in the fact that copper, although toxic, is also essential to mammalian life, as proven by its presence as a prosthetic element in cytochrome *c* oxidase,[1] tyrosinase,[2] lysyl oxidase[3] and several other specific copper-proteins and by well-defined pathologic effects caused by deficiency of copper.[4]

Yet, despite its essentiality, copper that is unincorporated into a specific copper-protein appears to play no physiologic role in man. Indeed, the toxicity of copper in patients with Wilson's disease is almost certainly a direct consequence of the fact that in vivo copper in excess of the body's requirements does not stimulate the synthesis of an equivalent excess of one or more apo-copper-proteins to incorporate, and thereby detoxify, the excess copper. As a result the latter is left free to combine with, and impair the function of, other molecules, such as proteins with sulfhydryl groups. It may have been the fact of copper's toxicity that forced the evolutionary process to use only protein-incorporated copper physiologically. There is normally almost no copper in vivo that is not bound to one or another specific copper-protein.

Another genetic abnormality of copper metabolism also provides evidence of the essentiality and toxicity of copper. Menkes' disease is an infantile, rare, fatal, and X-linked disorder of copper metabolism with characteristics of copper deficiency in that there are decreased concentrations of copper and ceruloplasmin in serum, of cytochrome *c* oxidase in liver and brain, and of lysyl oxidase in fibroblasts.[5, 6] Cultured fibroblasts from these infants are more susceptible than those from normal babies to the toxic effects of copper in the medium.[7–9] The disease (excellently reviewed by Danks[4]) seems to be caused by a defect in copper transport and not simply by impaired absorption of dietary copper, since neither oral nor parenteral administration of copper to an affected infant, no matter how early this is begun in the neonatal period, has proven to be effective therapy.

An autosomal recessive disorder of Bedlington terriers, characterized by copper toxicosis of the liver, has been studied in our laboratory for more than eight years.[10] We have also collaborated on an investigation of an inherited disturbance of copper metabolism in mice[11] and localized the excess hepatic copper found in the toad *Bufo marinus*[12] and the mute swan.[13] Each of these conditions shows some similarity to Wilson's disease—the liver disease of affected Bedlington terriers responds well to penicillamine therapy, for example—but there are significant pathologic, chemical, histochemical, ultrastructural and clinical differences between each and Wilson's disease.

We have not included a chapter on the natural history of Wilson's disease. There are several, which differ markedly from each other and which the reader can synthesize from portions of Chapters 4 and 7 through 13. Today these are, however, of historical rather than clinical interest, since they will be seen and recognized only in the very rare patient whose Wilson's disease is diagnosed but not treated. However, there are very different modes of presentation of Wilson's disease, as depicted in Figure 14–1, reflecting the variety of clinical courses the disease may take before a physician is consulted. For its correct diagnosis each mode requires somewhat different procedures and criteria.

There have been four international symposia devoted to Wilson's disease. The first, organized by Walshe and Cumings, was held in London in 1960[14]; the second, under the aegis of Yoshitoshi, in Tokyo in 1966[15]; the third, of which Boudin was chairman, in Paris in 1973[16]; and the fourth, arranged by Poch, in Buenos Aires in 1978.

In 1981 Owen published a volume on Wilson's disease[17] that has provided us with very helpful data, not the least of which is its comprehensive listing of references to the world's literature on this disorder.

REFERENCES

1. Nair, P. M., and Mason, H. S.: Reconstitution of cytochrome c oxidase from a copper-depleted enzyme and Cu^{I}. J. Biol. Chem. *242*:1406–1415, 1967.
2. Brown, F. C., and Ward, D. N.: Studies on mammalian tyrosinase. II. Chemical and physical properties of fractions purified by chromatography. Proc. Soc. Exp. Biol. Med. *100*:701–704, 1959.

3. Siegel, R. C., Pinnell, S. R., and Martin, G. R.: Cross-linking of collagen and elastin. Properties of lysyl oxidase. Biochemistry *9*:4486–4492, 1970.
4. Danks, D. M.: Copper deficiency in humans. *In* Biological Roles of Copper. Ciba Foundation Symposium 79, Excerpta Medica, Amsterdam, 1980, pp. 209–225.
5. Danks, D. M.: Copper transport and utilisation in Menkes' syndrome and in mottled mice. Inorg. Perspect. Biol. Med. *1*:73–100, 1977.
6. French, J.: X-chromosome linked copper malabsorption (X-cLCM). *In* Handbook of Clinical Neurology, Vol. 29. Ed. by Vinken, P. J., and Bruyn, G. W. North Holland Publishing Company, New York, 1977, pp. 297–304.
7. Beratis, N. G., Price, P., LaBadie, G., and Hirschhorn, K.: ^{64}Cu metabolism in Menkes and normal cultured skin fibroblasts. Pediatr. Res. 12:699–702, 1978.
8. Camakaris, J., Danks, D. M., Ackland, L., Cartwright, E., Borger, P., and Cotton, R. G. H.: Altered copper metabolism in cultured cells from human Menkes' syndrome and mottled mouse mutants. Biochem. Gen. *18*:117–131, 1980.
9. Chan, W.-Y., Garnica, A. D., and Rennert, O. M.: Cell culture studies of Menkes' kinky hair disease. Clin. Chim. Acta *88*:495–507, 1978.
10. Twedt, D. C., Sternlieb, I., and Gilbertson, S.: Clinical, morphologic and chemical studies on copper toxicosis of Bedlington terriers. J. Amer. Vet. Med. Assoc. *175*:269–275, 1979.
11. Biempica, L., Rauch, H., Goldfischer, S., Grushoff, P. S., and Sternlieb, I.: Inherited murine copper toxicosis. Hepatology *2*:722, 1982.
12. Goldfischer, S., Schiller, B., and Sternlieb, I.: Copper in hepatocyte lysosomes of the toad, *Bufo marinus L.* Nature *228*:172–173, 1970.
13. Molnar, J. J.: Copper storage in the liver of the wild mute swan (Cygnus olor). Arch. Pathol. Lab Med. (In press.)
14. Walshe, J. M., and Cumings, J. N., eds.: Wilson's Disease: Some Current Concepts. Blackwell, Oxford, 1961.
15. Bergsma, D., Scheinberg, I. H., and Sternlieb, I., eds.: Wilson's Disease. Birth Defects, Original Article Series, Vol. IV. The National Foundation—March of Dimes, New York, 1968.
16. Boudin, G., Pépin, B., and Hagueneau, M.: La maladie de Wilson. Nouv. Presse Méd. *3*:171–172, 1974.
17. Owen, C. A., Jr.: Wilson's Disease. Noyes Publications, Park Ridge, N.J., 1981.

CHAPTER 1

THE HISTORY OF WILSON'S DISEASE

In 1912 Samuel Alexander Kinnier Wilson, an American-born neurologist working in Great Britain, proposed the name *progressive lenticular degeneration* for a rare, familial, progressive and invariably fatal disease of young people manifested by involuntary movements, spasticity, dysphagia, dysarthria and, often, transitory mental symptoms. The disorder was characterized pathologically by bilateral, symmetrical softening in the lenticular nucleus and by cirrhosis of the liver. Wilson concluded his 211-page monograph, with a summary that is remarkable for his prediction that the "morbid agent is probably . . . a toxin . . . associated with the hepatic cirrhosis and . . . generated in connexion therewith."[1]

In an 1860 "Treatise on Diseases of the Liver," by Frerichs,[2] Wilson found a case history of a 10-year-old boy with clinical and pathologic findings virtually identical to those of the four cases he had observed personally as well as those of three patients of Homen's, two of Gowers' and one of Ormerod's, described about 1890.[1] Despite clinical and pathologic findings that were essentially the same as all of these, Wilson thought syphilis the etiology of Anton's case of "choreo-asthenic dementia with juvenile nodular cirrhosis of the liver" because of the "complete dementia" that has come to be recognized in the past 20 years as a devastating, if uncommon, complication of Wilson's disease.

In 1902 Kayser[3] (in a patient thought to have multiple sclerosis), and in 1903 Fleischer,[4] described the pigmented corneal rings now known by their names. Five years later Salus observed these rings in a patient diagnosed as suffering from multiple sclerosis[5] or "pseudosclerosis"—a term introduced by Westphal[6] in 1883 and by Strümpell[7] in 1898 to describe what is now considered to be Wilson's disease with predominantly tremulous neurologic manifestations.

In 1921 Hall noted that the inheritance of Wilson's disease might be as an autosomal recessive trait[8]—a hypothesis shown to be true 40 years later by Bearn.[9]

Rumpel was the first to find an excess of copper in the liver, in 1913,[10] a fact that does not seem to appear in the literature again until 1929, when Vogt,[11] and then Haurowitz[12] and Glazebrook,[13] reported excess copper in the brain and liver of patients. In 1934 Gerlach and Rohrschneider,[14] and, in 1936 Policard et al.,[15] showed that there was copper in the corneal region occupied by a Kayser-Fleischer ring.

In 1948 an unexpected experimental observation and a theoretical suggestion led to research that was to make Wilson's disease the first inherited and uniformly lethal disorder for which the signs and symptoms could be both virtually cured in the majority of clinically ill patients and prevented from becoming manifest in patients diagnosed while still asymptomatic.

The observation: Stimulated primarily by a paper by Bennetts and Chapman demonstrating a causal relation between copper deficiency and a fatal demyelinating disease of lambs,[16] Mandelbrote et al.[17] measured the urinary excretion of copper in five normal subjects, four patients with multiple sclerosis, and one each with Parkinson's disease, motor neurone disease, spinal cord tumor or Wilson's disease. In a two-hour period the patient with Wilson's disease excreted 41.7 mcg of copper, whereas none of the other twelve individuals excreted more than 18.0 mcg.

The suggestion: Cumings,[18] postulating an etiologic role for copper in Wilson's disease and aware of another finding reported in the paper of Mandelbrote's group—that 2,3-dimercaptopropanol (British Anti-Lewisite; BAL) increased the urinary excretion of copper, proposed that the use of this compound might be therapeutic.

In 1952 the diagnosis of Wilson's disease, on the basis of other than solely clinical criteria, became practical. One of us, learning that Wilson's disease seemed to be caused by excesses of copper in the central nervous system, began to measure the concentration of the copper-protein ceruloplasmin in the serum of these patients. Application of a spectrophotometric assay devised by Kominz, Oncley and Gurd demonstrated appreciable amounts of this protein in normal subjects but indicated that there was none at all in the serum of patients with Wilson's disease. Although the absence of a copper-protein seemed an illogical accompaniment of excess copper in various tissues, a quantitative immunochemical assay for ceruloplasmin, developed by Gitlin, confirmed that patients with Wilson's disease had a marked deficiency (though not generally an absence) of this protein,[19] a fact implicitly and almost simultaneously confirmed by Bearn and Kunkel.[20]

There is an ironic footnote to the discovery of the diagnostic significance of ceruloplasmin in Wilson's disease, in view of Holmberg's and Laurell's having been the first to purify, characterize, crystallize and name ceruloplasmin in four admirable papers published between 1947 and 1951.[21–24] Around 1948 Laurell had suspected that there might be abnormalities of ceruloplasmin in Wilson's disease but had found its concentration to be normal in the plasma of a patient who, he had been told, suffered from the illness. Unfortunately, the patient did *not* have Wilson's disease—a fact Laurell was not informed of until much later.

By the mid-1950s the wide and disparate variety of neurologic syndromes that had been described by Westphal,[6] Strümpell,[7] Wilson,[1]

Konovalov[25] and Boudin and Pépin[26] (among other clinicians) began to be recognized as merely differences in the clinical effects on the central nervous system of a single disorder of copper metabolism. When, at the same time, it became clear that all of these neurologic syndromes were uniquely characterized by deficiency of ceruloplasmin, excess deposits of copper in the brain and liver and the presence of Kayser-Fleischer rings, it was possible to confirm or exclude the diagnosis of Wilson's disease unequivocally, regardless of the neurologic symptomatology.

The fundamental and long-neglected roles of the liver in Wilson's disease, beginning with the discovery that ultrastructural[27] and structural[28] hepatic pathology always preceded damage to the central nervous system, as Wilson had intuitively believed, followed soon after Menghini developed a safe and simple technique of aspiration needle biopsy.[29]

In 1951 Denny-Brown and Porter,[30] as well as Cumings,[31] had independently confirmed the latter's prediction of the therapeutic efficacy of BAL. Unfortunately, the daily and indefinitely continued intramuscular injection of BAL was painful and impractical treatment for Wilson's disease. In 1955 Walshe, working at the Boston City Hospital, was asked to see a patient of Denny-Brown's with a failing liver. Having known and thought about the structure of penicillamine since finding it, several years previously, in the urine of patients receiving penicillin, Walshe was struck with the idea that the sulfhydryl group of this amino acid might make it capable of binding and excreting excess copper at least as readily as BAL and, since it should be orally administrable, painlessly. He obtained several grams of the compound and, suffering no ill effect when he swallowed some, gave it to a patient with Wilson's disease, in whom it produced a marked increase in urinary copper. Although he could obtain no more penicillamine, Walshe was able to buy about 50 grams of its thiazolidine derivative just before returning to his native England. There he converted the derivative compound to penicillamine and suggested to his father, the neurologist Sir Francis M. R. Walshe, that it be tested on one of his patients with Wilson's disease. Not only was it dramatically therapeutic in the ill young woman to whom it was given, but it proved to be a more effective cupriuretic agent than BAL on a weight basis.[32]

At the end of the 1950s, when it was clear that the long-term penicillamine treatment of patients with Wilson's disease was extraordinarily effective,[33] we began to treat asymptomatic individuals in whom the diagnosis of Wilson's disease was certain, in an effort to prevent the inexorable development of the disorder's signs and symptoms. In 1967 we submitted a manuscript to The New England Journal of Medicine with results of treating 53 asymptomatic patients that we believed showed that the continual daily administration of penicillamine could prevent clinically manifest Wilson's disease. The study did not, however, include a group of control subjects—asymptomatic patients who would not have received penicillamine—since we felt it would have been unjustified to withhold life-saving treatment from patients with a disease known for more than 50 years to be invariably fatal. (Our belief that this was the only course we could follow was further strengthened by the fact that 31 of the 36 asymptomatic patients in whom liver biopsy samples had been obtained had histologically evident fatty infiltration or cirrhosis.) In an editorial in the issue in which the paper finally appeared, Ingelfinger explained why he had overruled the recommendation of his editorial staff and consultants not to publish the article: "Sternlieb and Scheinberg's manuscript," he wrote, "has been seen by at least four clinicians conversant with liver disease, by two expert epidemiologists and by three biostatisticians. It has been discussed repeatedly and at length by the editorial staff; one editor even traveled to New York for a personal confrontation with one of the authors. Three major revisions were requested and acceded to without roiling passions. Yet the issue remained unresolved." After summarizing our case for publication, he continued, "The Journal's advisers in matters epidemiologic and statistical, however, remained unconvinced. Though sympathetic to the authors' dilemma as investigators of human illness, the referees' sympathy did not mitigate their criticism. They insisted with equal warmth the methods used did not prove the point." Then, citing several other authors who had urged application of techniques they had reported for diagnosing asymptomatic Wilson's disease, Ingelfinger concluded, "It was high time to publish the manuscript." The critical reader "must judge for himself."[34, 35]

In the weeks that followed, seven letters to the editor were published. Walshe[36] supported our procedure and conclusions; three letters were critical of us or the Journal[37–39]; two seemed to take the middle ground[40, 41]; and we responded in one.[42]

Because irreversible intolerance to penicillamine developed in a small proportion of patients with Wilson's disease, Walshe undertook to find an alternative means of treatment. By 1981, twelve years after its introduction, triethylene tetramine (trien, trientine, TETA) had been shown to be as effective, apparently, as penicillamine in the treatment of Wilson's disease.[43] In 1982 the U.S. Food and Drug Administration stated its intention to approve trien as an "orphan drug" for the treatment of patients with Wilson's disease who are irreversibly intolerant to penicillamine.[44]

REFERENCES

1. Wilson, S. A. K.: Progressive lenticular degeneration: A familial nervous disease associated with cirrhosis of the liver. Brain *34*:295–507, 1912.
2. Frerichs, F. T.: A Clinical Treatise on Diseases of the Liver, Vol. II. The New Sydenham Society, London, 1860, pp. 60–62.
3. Kayser, B.: Ueber einen Fall von angeborener grünlicher Verfärbung der Cornea. Klin. Mbl. Augenheilk. *40*:22–25, 1902.
4. Fleischer, B.: Zwei weitere Fälle von grünliche Verfärbung der Kornea. Klin. Mbl. Augenheilk. *41*:489–491, 1903.
5. Salus, R.: Grünliche Hornhautverfärbung bei multipler Sklerose. Med. Klin. *4*:495–497, 1908.
6. Westphal, C.: Ueber eine dem Bilde der cerebrospinalen grauen Degeneration ähnliche Erkrankung des centralen Nervensystems ohne anatomischen Befund, nebst einigen Bemerkungen über paradoxe Contraction. Arch. Psychiatr. Nervenkr. *14*:87–134, 1883
7. Strümpell, A.: Ueber die Westphal'sche Pseudosklerose und über diffuse Hirnsklerose, inbesondere bei Kindern. Dtsch. Z. Nervenheilk. *12*:115–149, 1898.
8. Hall, H. C.: La Dégénérescence Hépato-lenticulaire. Maladie de Wilson—Pseudosclérose. Masson, Paris, 1921.
9. Bearn, A. G.: A genetical analysis of thirty families with Wilson's disease (hepatolenticular degeneration). Ann. Hum. Genet. *24*:33–43, 1960.
10. Rumpel, A.: Ueber das Wesen und die Bedeutung der Leberveränderungen und der Pigmentierunen bei den damit verbundenen Fällen von Pseudosklerose, zugleich ein Beitrag zur Lehre von der Pseudosklerose (Westphal-Strümpell). Dtsch. Z. Nervenheilk. *49*:54–73, 1913.

11. Vogt, A.: Kupfer und Silber aufgespeichert in Auge, Leber, Milz und Nieren als Symptom der Pseudosklerose. Klin. Mbl. Augenheilk. *83*:417–419, 1929.
12. Haurowitz, F.: Ueber eine Anomalie des Kupferstoffwechsels. Hoppe-Seylers Z. Physiol. Chemie *190*:72–74, 1930.
13. Glazebrook, A. J.: Wilson's disease. Edinb. Med. J. *52*:83–87, 1945.
14. Gerlach, W., and Rohrschneider, W.: Besteht das Pigment des Kayser-Fleischerchen Hornhautringes aus Silber? Klin. Wschr. *13*:48–49, 1934.
15. Policard, A., Bonner, P., and Bonamour, G.: Etude histospectrographique de l'anneau cornéen de Kayser-Fleischer. C.R. Soc. Biol. (Paris) *122*:1120–1122, 1936.
16. Bennetts, H. W., and Chapman, F. E.: Copper deficiency in sheep in Western Australia: A preliminary account of the aetiology of enzootic ataxia of lambs and anaemia of ewes. Aust. Vet. J. *13*:138–149, 1937.
17. Mandelbrote, B. M., Stanier, M. W., Thompson, R. H. S., and Thruston, M. N.: Studies on copper metabolism in demyelinating diseases of the central nervous system. Brain *71*:212–228, 1948.
18. Cumings, J. N.: The copper and iron content of brain and liver in the normal and in hepato-lenticular degeneration. Brain *71*:410–415, 1948.
19. Scheinberg, I. H., and Gitlin, D.: Deficiency of ceruloplasmin in patients with hepatolenticular degeneration (Wilson's disease). Science *116*:484–485, 1952.
20. Bearn, A. G., and Kunkel, H. G.: Biochemical abnormalities in Wilson's disease. J. Clin. Invest. *31*:616, 1952.
21. Holmberg, C. G., and Laurell, C.-B.: Investigations in serum copper. I. Nature of serum copper and its relation to the iron-binding protein in human serum. Acta Chem. Scand. *1*:944–950, 1947.
22. Holmberg, C. G., and Laurell, C.-B.: Investigations in serum copper. II. Isolation of the copper containing protein, and a description of some of its properties. Acta Chem. Scand. *2*:550–556, 1948.
23. Holmberg, C. G., and Laurell, C.-B.: Investigations in serum copper. III. Caeruloplasmin as an enzyme. Acta Chem. Scand. *5*:476–480, 1951.
24. Holmberg, C. G., and Laurell, C.-B.: Investigations in serum copper. IV. Effect of different anions on the enzymatic activity of caeruloplasmin. Acta Chem. Scand. *5*:921–930, 1951.
25. Konovalov, N. V.: Hepatocerebral Dystrophy. Medgiz, Moscow, 1960.
26. Boudin, G., and Pépin, B.: Dégénérescence Hépatolenticulaire. Masson, Paris, 1959.
27. Sternlieb, I.: Mitochondrial and fatty changes in hepatocytes of patients with Wilson's disease. Gastroenterology *5*:354–367, 1968.
28. Sternlieb, I.: Evolution of the hepatic lesion in Wilson's disease. *In* Progress in Liver Diseases, Vol. IV. Ed. by Popper, H., and Schaffner, F. Grune & Stratton, New York, 1972, pp. 511–525.
29. Menghini, G.: One-second needle biopsy of the liver. Gastroenterology *35*:190–199, 1958.
30. Denny-Brown, D., and Porter, H.: The effect of BAL (2,3 dimercaptopropanol) on hepatolenticular degeneration (Wilson's disease). N. Engl. J. Med. *245*:917–925, 1951.
31. Cumings, J. N.: The effects of BAL in hepatolenticular degeneration. Brain *74*:10–22, 1951.
32. Walshe, J. M.: Penicillamine. A new oral therapy for Wilson's disease. Amer. J. Med. *21*:487–495, 1956.
33. Scheinberg, I. H., and Sternlieb, I.: Long term management of hepatolenticular degeneration (Wilson's disease). Amer. J. Med. *29*:316–333, 1960.
34. Ingelfinger, F., Editor's choice: Wilson's disease. N. Eng. J. Med. *278*:392–393, 1968.
35. Sternlieb, I., and Scheinberg, I. H.: Prevention of Wilson's disease in asymptomatic patients. N. Engl. J. Med. *278*:352–359, 1968.
36. Walshe, J. M.: Prophylactic use of penicillamine. N. Engl. J. Med. *278*:795–796, 1968.
37. Muench, H.: Prophylactic use of penicillamine. N. Engl. J. Med. *278*:796, 1968.
38. Chalmers, T. C.: Prophylactic treatment of Wilson's disease. New Engl. J. Med. *278*:910–911, 1968.
39. Fagan, T. J.: Prophylaxis of Wilson's disease (continued). New Engl. J. Med. *278*:1124–1125, 1968.
40. Kardinal, C. G.: Limitations of the scientific method. New Engl. J. Med. *278*:796, 1968.
41. Fagan, T. J.: Prophylaxis for Wilson's disease. New Engl. J. Med. *279*:271, 1968.
42. Sternlieb, I., and Scheinberg, I. H.: Prophylaxis of Wilson's disease (continued). New Engl. J. Med. *278*:1125, 1968.
43. Walshe, J. M.: Treatment of Wilson's disease with trientine (triethylene tetramine) dihydrochloride. Lancet *1*:643–647, 1982.
44. Hayes, A. H., Jr.: Triethylene tetramine dihydrochloride for treatment of penicillamine-intolerant patients with Wilson's disease; Invitation to submit new drug application. Fed. Reg. *47*:42175–42176, 1982.

CHAPTER 2

GENETICS

MODE OF INHERITANCE

In his original description Wilson[1] characterized the syndrome as familial. In 1921 Hall[2] analyzed the kinship of 68 patients, 34 of whom were related to at least one other patient by blood. Except in one kinship, all the related patients were siblings. It is clear that Hall was soon convinced that Wilson's disease was hereditary, and he concluded from his study that the underlying metabolic defect was transmitted by two different genes. His kinships, however, are totally consistent with transmission by a pair of a single autosomal recessive gene (WD gene), and his discussion indicates that he considered this mode, which he was the first to suggest, as only slightly less likely than his erroneous conclusion.

In 1950 André and van Bogaert reported a "high" percentage of consanguinity in 47 pairs of parents of 120 patients with Wilson's disease,[3] and Bearn later reported parental consanguinity in 14 of 30 affected families.[4] (One of Bearn's patients, F6, married to an unaffected first cousin who was shown to be a carrier,[5] had two daughters, F5 and E1, both of whom were found, in 1971, to have Wilson's disease.) In 1968 Arima and Sano reported that about half of 126 pairs of parents of 151 patients were consanguineous.[6] We have seen two families in which first cousins have had Wilson's disease, and Nordöy[7] has reported a third.

In another study of 206 individuals in five sibships, all of whom were related to one ancestral pair, 11 patients with Wilson's disease were identified, a prevalence of 5.3 per cent. Of the seven generations traced, members of the last four were available for study. Three patients were found in the fifth generation, and eight in the sixth. Four of the patients were in two sibships in which consanguinity was documented.[8]

Although Wilson's disease, as in the instances just cited, has been observed in successive generations, in the past 30 years we have seen only four instances of such an occurrence in which no evidence of consanguinity could be found: the daughter, D1, of a father, T3, with Wilson's disease and a healthy mother, shown by a test for heterozygosity[5] to be a carrier; the daughter of a mother with Wilson's disease, T1, and a healthy father who has not been tested for heterozygosity; a man and his nephew, M10, both with Wilson's disease; and a fourth family, which deserves special comment. In this family, the maternal aunt, M3, of a young man with Wilson's disease, C3, was sent to us when she was found to have multiple sclerosis at a university medical center. In view of her nephew's illness her local physician thought Wilson's disease might have been misdiagnosed as multiple sclerosis. The aunt was found, in fact, to have both multiple sclerosis (with optic neuritis and sensory changes) and Wilson's disease (with deficiency of ceruloplasmin, an abnormally elevated hepatic copper concentration, and characteristic histologic changes in the liver biopsy sample). As in the other three instances, no consanguinity could be established in this family, in either the parents or maternal grandparents of the young man who was the propositus.

These markedly excessive rates of consanguinity among parents of sons and daughters with Wilson's disease; the extreme rarity of affected members of successive generations in which there is no evidence of consanguinity; and the demonstration of the carrier state in the two healthy parents married to patients are further evidence (hardly necessary) of the autosomal recessive mode of inheritance of Wilson's disease. A disorder thus transmitted should affect 25 per cent of the children of heterozygous parents; whereas, if the WD gene were dominant, the disease would be expected to develop in 50 per cent of the children of a patient. Applying the Hardy-Weinberg formula to our data from 150 sibships, in which 252 of a total of 537 children had Wilson's disease, yields

$$(252-150)/(537-150) = 0.264$$

which does not differ significantly ($p > 0.05$) from the value of 0.25 expected for an autosomal recessive gene.

PREVALENCE AND GENE FREQUENCY

In 1968 we estimated (in reality, merely guessed from the fragmentary data available) that 1 in about 200,000 individuals in the general population had Wilson's disease.[9] From this ratio one can calculate the prevalence of the heterozygous carrier of the WD gene at about 1 in 224, with a corresponding gene frequency of about 1 in 448. This prevalence and gene frequency are considerably lower than the values we can calculate from three sets of data made available in the last 15 years.

1. In each of the eleven years from 1968 through 1978 the average number of deaths reported in the United States as being due to, or occurring in individuals with, Wilson's disease was 13.21 per million deaths,[10] a figure that, since the correct diagnosis of Wilson's disease is so infrequently suspected and made, is likely to be less than half of the true value.

2. In 1979, Bachmann and co-workers[11] in East Germany reported a WD gene frequency of 0.53 per cent, calculated from an accurately ascertained incidence of Wilson's disease of 29 in one million—about six times the prevalence rate we estimated in 1968. Because by 1979 the

TABLE 2–1. Ethnic and Geographic Origins of Patients with Wilson's Disease

American Indian
- *Cherokee

Arabs
- Iraqi[27]
- *Lebanese
- Libyan[28]
- *Moroccan
- *Palestinian[11b]
- *Tunisian[29]

*Argentinian[30]

Australian
- Aboriginal[31]
- Caucasian[32]

*Austrian[33]

Bashkirian[34]

Belgian[3, 35]

Blacks
- *American[13]
- *Haitian
- *Jamaican[36]
- Nigerian[37]
- Senegalese[38]
- S. African[39]
- *Trinidadian

*Brazilian[40]

*British[1, 4, 41]

Bulgarian[42]

Byelorussian[43]

*Canadian[14]

*Chilean[44]

*Chinese
- People's Republic[45]
- Taiwan[46]

Corsican[47]

*Czech[48]

Danish[2, 49]

*Druse[11b]

*Dutch[50]

Eskimo[51]

Estonian[52]

Finnish[53]

*French[54]

*German[11, 12, 55]

*Greek[56]

*Hungarian[57]

*Icelandic[58]

Indian
- Hindu[59]
- Muslim[59]
- Parsi[59]

Indonesian[60]

*Iranian[61, 62]

*Irish[13, 63]

*Italian
- Mainland[64]
- Sardinian[65]
- Sicilian[4]

Japanese[6]

Jews
- *Ashkenazi[11b, 13]
- *Iranian[11b]
- *Iraqi[11b]
- *N. African[11b]
- *Sephardic[11b]
- *Yemenite[11b]

Kirghizian[66]

*Lithuanian

Mexican[67]

*N. American[68-70]

Norwegian[71]

Pakistani[59]

*Philippine

*Polish[72]

*Portuguese

*Puerto Rican

Rumanian[73]

Russian[74, 75]

Scottish[76]

Serbian[77]

*Slovakian

Spanish[78]

Swedish[79]

Swiss[80]

*Thai[81]

Turkish[82]

*Ukrainian[83]

Uruguayan[84]

*Venezuelan

*Vietnamese[85]

*At least one patient from this group has been seen by the authors.

capabilities of correct diagnosis and effective treatment had been available for about 20 years, the prevalence rate was probably not much lower than the incidence rate. (The geographic distribution of the East German patients suggested that the latter was not significantly increased by consanguineous marriages.)

3. In 1981 Saito, from an analysis (which took account of consanguinity) of 289 Japanese families, each with at least one member with Wilson's disease, found the frequency of the disease to be 33 per million, and that of the gene to be 0.55 per cent.[11a]

From these data from widely separated populations and our knowledge that the WD gene is ubiquitous (Table 2–1) we conclude that the worldwide prevalence of patients with Wilson's disease is about 30 per million, with about one heterozygous carrier in each 90 persons. (This estimate of a gene frequency of approximately one in 180 has had to be based on knowledge of the prevalence or incidence of the disease, since, as discussed below, the heterozygous carrier of one WD gene can be neither accurately nor practically detected.)

Where there is a significant degree of consanguinity in a population, the prevalence of patients and the frequency of the abnormal gene is likely to be higher than in nonconsanguineous areas. This is true, for example, of certain Arab, Druse, Iranian and Yemenite Jewish communities.[11b]

GENE EXPRESSION

Although there are often similarities in the age of onset and clinical manifestations of Wilson's disease among affected siblings,[6, 12] we have frequently seen differences in symptomatology, as well as in biochemical findings, among patient-siblings. A brother, M11, and a sister, M12, for example, manifested solely disease of the liver, and both died without any neurologic disturbance. But a second sister, M13, had severe, incapacitating neurologic disturbances and no overt clinical evidence of liver affection. Affected siblings of consanguineous marriages appear to differ from each other just as much as other patient-siblings. The only siblings of whom we are aware who exhibited virtually identical clinical and biochemical findings of Wilson's disease are a pair of uniovular twins, R5 and R6.[13]

These variations between affected siblings are due to a "genetic basis"[14] only in the trivial sense that they are attributable to the effects of the entire genome on the expression of the abnormal pair of WD genes. This seems a reasonable explanation, as well, for the earlier onset and increased severity of the disease noted in certain Arab[11b] and Japanese[6] patients.

WD GENE MARKERS

A deficiency of ceruloplasmin in serum, exhibited by about 95 per cent of patients with Wilson's disease, is the only generally accepted genetic marker of this disorder. It has, however, never been demonstrated

TABLE 2–2. Distribution of Concentrations of Ceruloplasmin in the Serum of 88 Heterozygous Carriers

CERULOPLASMIN (mg/dl)	PATIENTS *Number*	*Per Cent*
0	0	0
1– 4.9	1	1.1
5– 9.8	1	1.1
10–14.9	2	2.3
15–19.9	14	15.9
>20	70	79.6
	88	100.0

that this protein is the primary gene product of the normal allele of the WD gene: approximately 25 per cent of patients with Wilson's disease have no detectable ceruloplasmin; all of the others have some of the protein; and about 5 per cent exhibit normal levels of ceruloplasmin. Reports of structural abnormalities in patients' ceruloplasmin (see Chapter 3) have not been confirmed.

About 20 per cent of heterozygotes have deficiency of ceruloplasmin; a very few heterozygotes have very little detectable ceruloplasmin (Table 2–2).

Two groups of workers believe that fingerprint characteristics (palmar dermatoglyphics) can provide a genetic marker for Wilson's disease,[15–17] but two other reports could not confirm this finding.[18, 19] One published study and our own studies on two families could reveal no correlation of patients with Wilson's disease and HLA types.[20]

In a recent study of a different kind, cultured fibroblasts from the skin of patients with Wilson's disease had approximately three times the concentration of intracellular copper found in cultures from control subjects, suggesting that the genetic defect underlying this disorder is expressed in these cells.[21]

A hypothesis that the WD gene is a mutant of a single regulator gene that impairs both ceruloplasmin synthesis and biliary copper excretion[22] is discussed in Chapter 4.

DETECTION OF THE HETEROZYGOUS CARRIER OF THE WD GENE

Although the unequivocal confirmation or exclusion of the diagnosis of Wilson's disease is almost always feasible, the detection of the heterozygous carrier of one WD gene is much less reliable. All the tests described[5, 23–26] depend upon measuring radiocopper's bodily distribution, incorporation into ceruloplasmin or urinary excretion, or on a combination of these measurements. Because it has probably been applied to larger groups than any other, the statistical degree of certainty of the empirical test we devised and validated more than 20 years ago is at least as good, in our opinion, as any other.[5] The only change we have introduced in the procedure given in 1961 is the use of ginger ale or fruit juice in place of milk as the beverage in which the copper is ingested. We found, fortuitously, that absorption of copper from milk is inhibited and variable from subject to subject because of the metal's entrapment in the gastric precipitate of lactoglobulin.

REFERENCES

1. Wilson, S. A. K.: Progressive lenticular degeneration: A familial nervous disease associated with cirrhosis of the liver. Brain *34*:295–507, 1912.
2. Hall, H. C.: La Dégénérescence Hépato-lenticulaire. Maladie de Wilson—Pseudosclérose. Masson, Paris, 1921, p. 361.
3. André, M. J., and van Bogaert, L.: L'hérédité dans la dégénérescence hépatolenticulaire et le problème des rapports intrinsèques de la pseudosclérose de Westphal-Strümpell et de la maladie de Wilson. La situation nosologique de l'"Abdominal Wilson" de Kehrer au sein de la DHL. Encéphale *39*:1–54, 1950.
4. Bearn, A. G.: A genetical analysis of thirty families with Wilson's disease (hepatolenticular degeneration). Ann. Hum. Genet. *24*:33–43, 1960.
5. Sternlieb, I., Morell, A. G., Bauer, C. D., Combes, B., deBobes-Sternberg, S., and Scheinberg, I. H.: Detection of the heterozygous carrier of the Wilson's disease gene. J. Clin. Invest. *40*:707–715, 1961.
6. Arima, M., and Sano, I.: Genetic studies of Wilson's disease in Japan. *In* Wilson's Disease. Birth Defects, Original Article Series, Vol. VI. Ed. by Bergsma, D., Scheinberg, I. H., and Sternlieb, I. The National Foundation—March of Dimes, New York, 1968, pp. 54–63.
7. Nordöy, A.: Wilson's disease. Acta Med. Scand. *172*:445–449, 1962.
8. Melendez, M. G., Williams, D. M., Baty, B., and Cartwright, G. E.: Clinical studies of a large family with Wilson's disease. South. Med. J. *73*:607–610, 1980.
9. Sternlieb, I., and Scheinberg, I. H.: Prevention of Wilson's disease in asymptomatic patients. N. Engl. J. Med. *278*:352–359, 1968.
10. Vital Statistics of the United States. Vol. II, Mortality; Part A, Tables 1–23, 1968–1978; and Dr. Harry M. Rosenberg (personal communication).
11. Bachmann, H., Lössner, J., Gruss, B., and Ruchholtz, U.: Die Epidemiologie der Wilsonschen Erkrankung in der DDR und die derzeitige Problematik einer populationgenetischen Bearbeitung. Psychiat. Neurol Med. Psychol. (Leipzig) *31*:393–400, 1979.

11a. Saito, T.: An assessment of efficiency in potential screening for Wilson's disease. J. Epidemiol. Comm. Health *35*:274–280, 1981.

11b. Passwell, J., Adam, A., Garfinkel, D., Streifler, M., and Cohen, B. E.: Heterogeneity of Wilson's disease in Israel. Isr. J. Med. Sci. *13*:15–19, 1977.

12. Bachmann, H. V., Lössner, J., Biesold, D., and Gunther, K.: Genetische Studien zur Wilsonschen Erkrankung in der DDR und Konsequenzen für Diagnostik und Beratung. Dtsch. Gesundh-Wesen *35*:1052–1055, 1980.
13. Bearn, A. G., and Kunkel, H. G.: Abnormalities of copper metabolism in Wilson's disease and their relationship to the aminoaciduria. J. Clin. Invest. *33*:400–409, 1954.
14. Wilson-Cox, D., Fraser, F. C., and Sass-Kortsak, A.: A genetic study of Wilson's disease: evidence for heterogeneity. Amer. J. Human. Genet. *24*:646–666, 1972.
15. Hodges, R. E., and Simon, J. R.: Relationship between fingerprint patterns and Wilson's disease. J. Lab. Clin. Med. *60*:629–640, 1962.
16. Vormittag, W., Weninger, M., Willvonseder, R., and Wewalka, F.: Hautleistenverlauf bei Homo- und Heterozygotie für Morbus Wilson (Hepatolentikuläre Degeneration). Hum. Genet. *31*:211–218, 1976.
17. Vormittag, W., Weninger, M., and Hayek, H.: Zur Beziehung zwischen Hautleistenverlauf und Morbus Wilson. Hum. Genet. *18*:337–340, 1973.
18. Grosse, R.: Dermatoglyphic analysis as a diagnostic tool in Wilson's disease? Hum. Genet. *28*:281–284, 1975.
19. David, T. J., and Ajdukiewicz, A. B.: Palmar dermatoglyphs in Wilson's disease. Brit. Med. J. *3*:825–826, 1972.
20. Tabacchi, P. L., Bordini, G., Barboni, F., Corazza, G. R., and Gasbarrini, G.: Inheritance of HLA antigens in a family with Wilson's disease. *In* Histocompatibility Testing, Report of the 7th Histocompatibility Workshop. Oxford, Ed. by Bodmer, W. F. Munksgaard, Copenhagen, 1977, p. 484.
21. Chan, W. Y., Cushing, W., Coffman, M. A., and Rennert, O. M.: Genetic expression of Wilson's disease in cell culture: a diagnostic marker. Science *208*:299–300, 1980.
22. Epstein, O., and Sherlock, S.: Is Wilson's disease caused by a controller gene mutation resulting in perpetuation of the fetal mode of copper metabolism? Lancet *1*:303–305, 1981.
23. Wesch, H., Przuntek, H., and Feist, D.: Morbus Wilson. Dtsch. Med. Wschr. *105*:483–488, 1980.
24. Sternlieb, I., and Scheinberg, I. H.: Radiocopper in diagnosing liver disease. Semin. Nucl. Med. *2*:176–188, 1972.

25. Tauxe, W. N., Goldstein, N. P., Randall, R. V., and Gross, J. B.: Radiocopper studies in patients with Wilson's disease and their relatives. Amer. J. Med. *41*:375–380, 1966.
26. Sternlieb, I., Morell, A. G., and Scheinberg, I. H.: Homozygosity and heterozygosity in Wilson's disease. *In* Wilson's Disease: Some Current Concepts. Ed. by Walshe, J. M., and Cumings, J. N. Blackwell, Oxford, 1961, pp. 133–140.
27. Bakos, S. N.: Polyarthritis associated with Wilson's disease. Arch. Dis. Child. *54*:985, 1979.
28. Sherlock, S. Personal communication.
29. Hamza, B., and el-Kamel, M.: Two cases of Wilson's disease diagnosed at the infra-clinical stage. Prolonged, early treatment using penicillamine. Result. Tunis Méd. *52*:29–31, 1974.
30. Thomson, A. F., Bardeci, C. A., and Katz, S.: Degeneracion Hépato-Lenticular. Arch. Fund. Roux-Ocefa *1*:273–282, 1967.
31. Gollan, J. L., Hicks, E. P., and Gordon, J. V.: Hepatolenticular degeneration (Wilson's disease) in an Australian aboriginal. Med. J. Austral. *2*:1197–1199, 1970.
32. Danks, D. M., and Stevens, B. J.: Diagnosis of Wilson's disease in children with liver disease. A report of two families. Lancet *1*:22–25, 1969.
33. Hayek, H. W., Knoll, E., and Widhalm, S.: Uber das organische Psychosyndrom bei Morbus Wilson (Langzeitbeobachtung mit psychologischen Testergebnissen bei 4 Patienten unter D-penicillamin-therapie). Mschr. Kinderheilk. *121*:679–683, 1973.
34. Magzhanov, R. V., Pertsev, G. S., and Trishna, N. I.: Concerning diagnosis of heterozygotic carrying of the hepatocerebral dystrophy gene. Sovetskaia Meditsina *7*:28–30, 1979.
35. Bollen, J., Sevrynck, D., Proesmans, W., Fevery, J., and De Groote, J.: Ziekte van Wilson. Beschrijving van enkele gevallen. Tijdschr. Gastro-enterologie *3*:129–139, 1978.
36. Miller, G. J., and Persaud, V.: Hereditary hepatolenticular degeneration (Wilson's disease). Report on the first case in Jamaica. Trop. Geogr. Med. *20*:225–232, 1968.
37. Longe, A. C., Glew, R. H., and Omene, J. A.: Wilson's disease. Report of a case in a Nigerian. Arch. Neurol. *39*:129–130, 1982.
38. Dumas, M., Girard, P.-L., Jacquin-Cotton, L., and Konaté, S.: Premier cas de maladie de Wilson au Sénégal. Bull. Soc. Med. Afr. Noire lgue fr. *15*:96–99, 1970.
39. Van Der Merwe, C. F., and Padayatchi, P.: Wilsonse siekte in 'n swart Pasient. Gevalbespreking en kort Literatuuroorsig. S. Afr. Med. J. *54*:616–618, 1978.
40. Canelas, H. M., Escalente, O. D., DeJorge, F. B., and Roche-Quintao, E. C.: Hepatolenticular degeneration. Clinical and biochemical study of three cases. Arq. Neuro/Psiq. *21*:229–250, 1963.
41. Walshe, J. M.: Wilson's disease (hepatolenticular degeneration). *In* Handbook of Clinical Neurology. Metabolic and Deficiency Diseases of the Nervous System, Vol. 27, Part I. Ed. by Vinken, P. J., Bruyn, G. W., and Klawans, H. L. American Elsevier Publishing Co., New York, 1976, pp. 379–414.
42. Brailski, Chr., Kolarski, V., and Krastev, I.: Untersuchungen über die hepatolentikuläre Degeneration und Ergebnisse ihrer Dauerbehandlung. Dtsch. Z. Verdau Stoffwechselkr. *30*:35–42, 1970.
43. Grigorieva, N. K.: Psychological manifestations in children with hepatolenticular degeneration. Z. Nevropatol. Psikh. *72*:1568–1570, 1972.
44. Tocornal, J. A., Monckeberg, F., Etchart, M., and Montero, E.: Enfermedad de Wilson (Degeneracion hepatolenticular). Rev. Chilena Med. 839–841, 1960.
45. Xu, X. H., Yang, B. X., and Feng, Y. K.: Wilson's disease (hepatolenticular degeneration). Clinical analysis of 80 cases. Chin. Med. J. *94*:673–678, 1981.
46. Strickland, G. T., Frommer, D., Leu, M.-L., Pollard, R., Sherlock, S., and Cumings, J. N.: Wilson's disease in the United Kingdom and Taiwan. I. General characteristics of 142 cases and prognosis. II. A genetic analysis of 88 cases. Quart. J. Med. *42*:619–638, 1973.
47. Bérard-Badier, M., Löwenthal, A., Bernard, R., Payan, H., and Gastaut, H.: Dégénérescence hépato-lenticulaire. Etude anatomo-clinique, électroencéphalographique et biochimique à propos de trois cas dont deux jumeaux. Psychiat. Neurol. (Basel) *140*:445–475, 1960.
48. Hauftovà, D., Hartl, J., Seidlova, V., Ruzickova, R., Kubena, K., and Slavicek, J.: Penicillamine in the treatment of Wilson's disease. Vnitr. lek. *16*:337–343, 1970.
49. Plum, L., Jensen, K. G., and Palm, L.: Hepatolenticular degeneration. Report of a case and investigation of the family. Ugeskr. Laeg. *129*:583–586, 1967.
50. Plooj, M., van der Meer, J., and Kaag, A.: Enige onderzoekingen bij hepatolenticulaire degeneratie. Ned. T. Geneesk. *103*:200–204, 1959.
51. Fog-Poulsen, M.: Degeneratio hepatolenticularis hos en Gronlaender. Ugeskr. Laeg. *111*:10–11, 1949.
52. Willemi, K.: Die Veränderungen in der Hirnrinde und in den Stammganglien nach experimenteller Leberschädigung. Folia Neuropathol. Estonia *2*:109–143, 1924.
53. Karma, A.: Ophthalmologic and genetic aspects of Wilson's disease (hepatolenticular degeneration). Acta Ophthalmologica Kbh. *51*:383–389, 1973.
54. Boudin, G., and Pépin, G.: Dégénérescence Hépato-Lenticulaire. Masson, Paris, 1959.
55. Lange, J.: Long term treatment of Wilson's disease with D-penicillamine. *In* Wilson's Disease. Birth Defects, Original Article Series, Vol. IV. Ed. by Bergsma, D., Scheinberg, I. H., and Sternlieb, I. The National Foundation—March of Dimes, New York, 1968, pp. 130–133.
56. Kaklamanis, P., and Spengos, M.: Osteoarticular changes and synovial biopsy findings in Wilson's disease. Ann. Rheum. Dis. *32*:422–427, 1973.
57. Gacs, J., Kerekes, E., and Wurfer, B.: Die Wilsonsche Krankheit (Degeneratio hepatolenticularis). Wiener Zschr. Inn. Med. *6*:226–233, 1965.

58. Gudmundsson, K. R.: Prevalence and occurrence of some rare neurological diseases in Iceland. Acta Neurol. Scand. *45*:114–118, 1969.
59. Dastur, D. K., Manghani, D. K., and Wadia, N. H.: Wilson's disease in India. I. Geographic, genetic, and clinical aspects in 16 families. Neurology *18*:21–31, 1968.
60. Cohen, A. J., and Tamaela, L.: Een geval van hepato-lenticulaire Degeneratie. Geneesk. Tijdschr. v. Ned.-Indie *68*:269–277, 1928.
61. Korourian, M., and Djavadi, A.: The biochemical diagnosis of Wilson's disease in Iran. Arch. Inst. Razi. *21*:35–38, 1969.
62. Gharib, M., Moazzami, R., and Behbakht, G. H.: Wilson's disease. Report of patient with osseous manifestations. Clin. Pediat. *9*:625–626, 1970.
63. Warnock, C. G.: Wilson's disease in general practice. *In* Wilson's Disease: Some Current Concepts. Ed. by Walshe, J. M., and Cumings, J. N., Blackwell, Oxford, 1961, pp. 205–210.
64. Berio, A., Vento, R., and DiStefano, A.: Favorable results with an association of L-dopa and amantadine added to penicillamine in the treatment of Wilson's disease. Minerva Pediatr. *19*:807–813, 1973.
65. Giagheddu, M., and Chessa-Perle, E.: Studio dell'attività rame-ossidasica serica in otto famiglie colpite da malattia di Strumpell-Wilson (Degenerazione epato-lenticulare). Sist. Nerv. *4*:237–352, 1961.
66. Belekova, R. B.: Konovalov-Wilson's disease. Zdravookhr. Kirg. *2*:51–53, 1976.
67. Gonzalez-Angulo, A., Trevino, N., Perches, A., and Zavala, B. J.: Wilson's disease: An electron microscope study. Bol. Inst. Estud. Med. Biol. *23*:155–168, 1965.
68. Cartwright, G. E., Hodges, R. E., Gubler, C. J., Mahoney, J. P., Daum, K., Wintrobe, M. M., and Bean, W. B.: Studies on copper metabolism. XIII. Hepatolenticular degeneration. J. Clin. Invest. *33*:1487–1501, 1954.
69. Sternlieb, I., and Scheinberg, I. H.: The prevention of Wilson's disease in asymptomatic patients. N. Engl. J. Med. *278*:352–359, 1968.
70. Goldstein, N. P., and Gross, J. B.: Treatment of Wilson's disease. *In* Clinical Neuropharmacology, Vol. 2. Ed. by Klawans, H. L. Raven Press, New York, 1977, pp. 99–112.
71. Lygren, T., Sorensen, E. W., and Bernhardsen, A.: Hepatolenticular degeneration (Wilson's disease). A case diagnosed biochemically before clinical manifestations. Lancet *1*:276–277, 1959.
72. Wald, I., and Niewiarowska, M.: Etude clinique et biologique de la coagulation et de la fibrinolyse dans les 12 cas de dégénérescence hépatolenticulaire. Sang. *30*:560–566, 1959.
73. Ionasescu, V., Costa-Foru, D., Rosianu, C., and Luca, N.: Biochemical investigations and clinical correlation in hepatolenticular degeneration. Rev. Roumaine Neurol. *1*:229–239, 1964.
74. Konovalov, N. V.: Hepatocerebral Dystrophy. Medgiz, Moscow, 1960.
75. Bondarchuk, A. N., Vakharlovsky, V. G., Kliorin, A. I., Melynecheva, L. A., Shavlovsky, M. M., Yakovkina, E. O., and Neifakh, S. A.: Early diagnosis of hepatocellular degeneration in children. Vopr. Okhr. Mater. Detsva (Moscow) *20*:28–33, 1975.
76. Morgan, H. G., Stewart, W. K., Lowe, K. G., Stowers, J. M., and Johnstone, J. H.: Wilson's disease and the Fanconi syndrome. Quart. J. Med. *31*:361, 384, 1962.
77. Aksamija-Rizvic, B.: Wilson's disease treated with penicillamine. Lij. Vjes. *98*:430–431, 1976.
78. Guardia, J., Barcardi, R., Martinez-Vazquez, J. M., Torruella, M., Fiol, C., Schwartz, S., Buendia, E., Rona, V., and Tornos, J.: Enfermedad de Wilson de localization exclusivamente hepatica. (Estudio de una familia.) Rev. Clin. Esp. *129*:463–468, 1973.
79. Nyberg, P., Gottfries, C.-G., Holmgren, G., Persson, S., Roos, B.-E., and Winblad, B.: Advanced catecholaminergic disturbances in the brain in a case of Wilson's disease. Arch. Neurol. Scand. *65*:71–75, 1982.
80. Tschumi, A., Colombo, J. P., and Moser, H.: Die Wilsonsche Krankheit in der Schweiz. Klinische genetische und biochimische Untersuchungen. Schweiz. Med. Wschr. *103*:89–95, 1973.
81. Ishizaki, T., Chitanondh, H., and Laksanavicharn, U.: Wilson's disease. Clinicopathologic report of 4 cases. J. Med. Assoc. Thailand *51*:419–443, 1968.
82. Aksoy, M., Camli, N., Dilsen, G., Kocak, N., Erdem, S., Ozdogan, E., Dincol, K., and Dincol, G.: Osteoarticular pains and changes in Wilson's disease. A radiological study of fourteen patients in nine Turkish families. Acta Hepato-Gastroenterol. *22*:164–170, 1975.
83. Leschtschenko, G. D.: Beiträge zum Studium der Pseudosklerose. Arch. Psychiatr. Nervenkrank. *75*:392–400, 1925.
84. Ruggia, R., Maslenikov, O., Estable-Puig, C., Ferrer, J., Bidegain, S., Negro, R. C., Temesio, N., Perez-Scremini, A., and Soto, J. A.: Degeneracion hepatolenticular. Enfermedad de Wilson. Nuevo aporte a la casuistica. Acta Neurol. Latinoamer. *12*:130–141, 1966.
85. Huong, B. Q., Bezon, A. G., Thong, N. N.: Dégénérescence hépato-lenticulare au Vietnam. Une étude statistique, clinique, évolutive échelonnée sur 10 ans concernant 8 cas personnels. Presse Méd. *78*:1147–1150, 1970.

CHAPTER 3

CERULOPLASMIN

In Wilson's disease no significant abnormality has been described in any human copper-protein except ceruloplasmin, a protein first characterized by Holmberg and Laurell.[1–4] Marked deficiency of ceruloplasmin is seen in more than 95 per cent of patients. With one exception discussed below, the few other conditions in which ceruloplasmin deficiency may be seen—the neonatal state,[5] Menkes' disease,[6] kwashiorkor,[7] marasmus,[8] nephrotic syndrome,[9] protein-losing enteropathy,[10] tropical and non-tropical sprue,[11, 12] severe copper deficiency[13, 14] and severe hepatic insufficiency[15]—are readily distinguishable from Wilson's disease. This unique diagnostic significance of ceruloplasmin makes it worthwhile to summarize current information about it critically, emphasizing those aspects that may bear on its functional relationship to Wilson's disease.

GENERAL CHEMICAL AND PHYSICAL PROPERTIES

Ceruloplasmin—an intensely blue, alpha-2-globulin with a molecular weight of about 132,000[15a, 15b, 16–18]—contains 0.3 per cent copper and 8 per cent carbohydrate and is normally present in a concentration of 20 to 40 mg/dl of human plasma.[18] It is a single-chain polypeptide whose amino acid composition has been determined[19] (Table 3–1) and whose amino acid sequence is known for more than half of the protein.[17, 20]

Ceruloplasmin exhibits varying degrees of oxidase activity toward certain aromatic amines and phenols, cysteine, the ferrous ion and ascorbic acid,[21-24] although this activity has not been shown to be of indubitable physiologic or pathologic significance in man.

Of the six prosthetic copper atoms in each molecule, two are cupric, blue and capable of being reduced and re-oxidized; one is cupric, not blue and believed to be capable of binding anions; two are thought to be a spin-coupled pair of cupric ions; and one is characterized only as being required by the copper content of the molecule.[16] Only the first three exhibit electron paramagnetic resonance.

TABLE 3–1. Amino Acid Composition of Human Ceruloplasmin[14]

Amino Acid	Number of Residues
Lysine	74.4
Histidine	45.2
Arginine	40.3
Aspartic acid	118.4
Threonine	77.0
Serine	68.0
Glutamic acid	120.9
Proline	49.6
Glycine	78.4
Alanine	49.5
Half-cystine	13.8
Valine	60.0
Methionine	23.1
Isoleucine	51.1
Leucine	69.4
Tyrosine	63.3
Phenylalanine	48.2
Tryptophane	14.3
Sum of residues	1065

Each molecule of ceruloplasmin contains one triantennary and two biantennary oligosaccharide chains of mannose, *N*-acetyl glucosamine, galactose and sialic acid covalently linked to an asparagine residue.[25]

The validity of using in vitro and in vivo radiocopper-labeled ceruloplasmin to measure the intravascular survival of the protein depends on three observations indicating that in humans ceruloplasmin-copper does not appear to exchange to any significant degree with other pools of copper in vivo. First, when ^{67}copper-labeled ceruloplasmin was injected intravenously into two aceruloplasminemic patients with Wilson's disease, G6 and S16, there was no difference in the survival of the protein determined either from the rate of decrease, in serum, of the concentration of ^{67}copper or of the specific oxidase activity of ceruloplasmin.[26] Second, there was no significant difference between the half-life of ^{67}copper-labeled ceruloplasmin[26] and that of ^{131}iodine-labeled ceruloplasmin,[27] which was injected into control subjects, indicating that copper is not released from the protein in the circulation. Finally, the rate of incorporation of radiocopper into ceruloplasmin in vivo doubled when exogenous stimulation doubled the rate of synthesis of ceruloplasmin. But the rate of incorporation was unchanged when the serum concentration of this protein was almost tripled passively by intravenous infusion of concentrated human ceruloplasmin, observations also showing that the infused circulating ceruloplasmin exchanged none of its copper.[26]

However, Campbell et al.[28] have concluded that such exchange of copper occurs in vivo in the rat, in which animal ceruloplasmin-copper "turns over more rapidly than the protein moiety," implying that "at least some of the copper on this molecule is removed and replaced" in vivo. We believe these results are erroneous, since the preparations of ^{67}copper-labeled ceruloplasmin used appear to have been significantly contaminated with non–ceruloplasmin-^{67}copper, as a result of which the physiologic half-life of labeled ceruloplasmin found by these investigators was more than an order of magnitude shorter than that reported in published data.[29]

Descriptions of other chemical and physical properties of ceruloplasmin are given in two reviews.[18, 22]

EFFECTS OF PHYSIOLOGIC AND PATHOLOGIC FACTORS ON THE CONCENTRATION OF CERULOPLASMIN

The concentration of ceruloplasmin—generally between 20 and 40 mg/dl of plasma or serum in the normal adult—rises, occasionally reaching 100 mg/dl, during the latter stages of pregnancy; when estrogens are administered; and in a number of pathologic states that include infection, certain active non-Wilsonian liver diseases, rheumatoid arthritis, some neoplastic disorders and a number of conditions associated with inflammatory or necrotic changes.[5, 30] Although less than 20 mg/dl may be seen in the conditions named in the first paragraph of this chapter, the only specific diagnostic significance attaching to abnormal concentrations of ceruloplasmin, at least in humans, is its hereditary deficiency in Wilson's disease (Table 3–2) and Menkes' syndrome.[6]

Hereditary deficiency of ceruloplasmin is not sufficient to confirm a diagnosis of Wilson's disease. About 20 per cent of heterozygotes may exhibit less than 20 mg/dl of ceruloplasmin,[31] as shown in Table 2–2. Moreover, it is possible that another mutant gene may be associated with hypoceruloplasminemia without excessive copper retention.[32] Indeed, as is apparent from Table 3–2, ceruloplasmin deficiency is not even necessary for the diagnosis, since about 5 per cent of patients—not pregnant, not receiving estrogens, or not suffering from any of the disorders listed in the preceding paragraph—have normal concentrations of ceruloplasmin in the 20 to 30 mg/dl range.

Table 3–3 and Fig. 3–1 illustrate the ways in which the concentration of ceruloplasmin may change in a patient with Wilson's disease during treatment with penicillamine. The concentration may fall (Group A), may

TABLE 3–2. Distribution of Pretreatment Concentrations of Ceruloplasmin in Serum of Patients with Wilson's Disease

Ceruloplasmin (mg/dl)	Gibbs and Walshe[31]*		Sass-Kortsak and Bearn[55]†		Authors' Patients‡	
	n	%	n	%	n	%
<5	48	64	136	59	190	52
5–20	23	31	83	36	162	44
>20	4	5	11	5	15	4
	75	100	230	100	367	100

*Determined by quantitative assay of each serum's oxidase activity toward dimethyl *p*-phenylenediamine, calibrated against solutions of purified ceruloplasmin.

†Method of assay not specified.

‡Determined by quantitative assay of each serum's oxidase activity toward *p*-phenylenediamine, calibrated against both solutions of purified ceruloplasmin in serum and sera of known ceruloplasmin-copper concentrations.

TABLE 3–3. Concentration of Serum Ceruloplasmin During Penicillamine Treatment of Four Groups of Patients with Wilson's Disease

Group	No.	Years of Treatment (mean)	Ceruloplasmin Before Treatment (mean ± S.D.) (mg/dl)	Ceruloplasmin After Treatment (mean ± S.D.) (mg/dl)
A	12	10.3	15.7 ± 9.3	6.5 ± 6.4
B	12	11.9	2.0	2.0
C	12	13.9	5.1 ± 4.1	18.4 ± 4.1
D	3	6.0	22.4 ± 2.9	25.3 ± 5.4

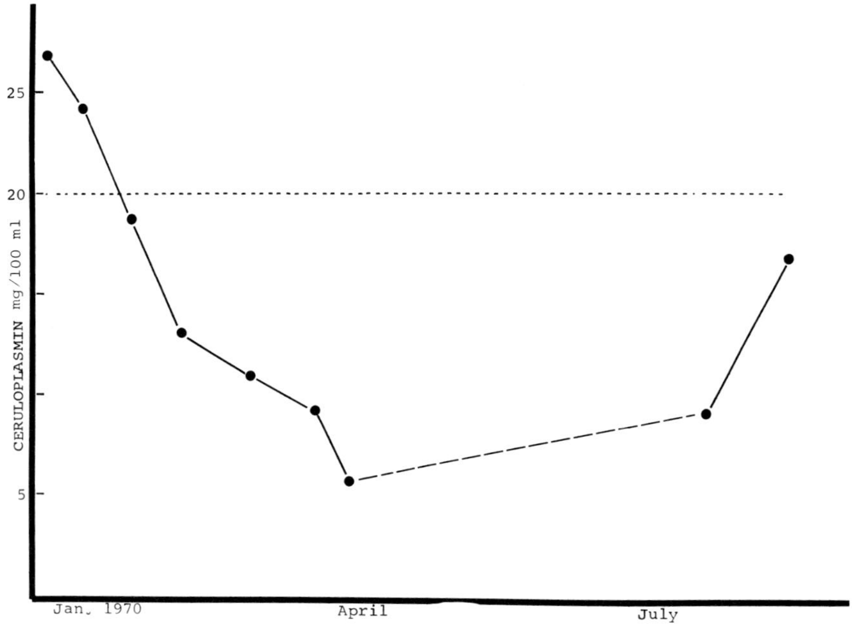

Figure 3–1. Variations in serum ceruloplasmin concentrations in patient R4 over an eight-month period, during which improvement in her liver disease was accompanied by a fall in serum ceruloplasmin to levels characteristic of patients with Wilson's disease. The lower limit of the normal range of serum ceruloplasmin concentration (20 mg/dl) is indicated. (From Sternlieb, I., and Scheinberg, I.. H.: Ann. Int. Med. *76*:59–64, 1972; with permission of the Annals of Internal Medicine).

not change (Group B), or may rise (Group C). Even more puzzling are the very few patients whose pretreatment normal concentrations of ceruloplasmin remain so during therapy (Group D). We have been unable to correlate any of these types of responses with any physiologic, pharmacologic or pathologic factor or with therapeutic results. The concentration of ceruloplasmin is of diagnostic, but not prognostic, value.

DEFICIENCY OF CERULOPLASMIN IN WILSON'S DISEASE

There are at least three possible mechanisms—none proven—by which deficiency of ceruloplasmin may be caused in Wilson's disease.

1. As a result of qualitative differences. In 1961 Hirschman et al.[33] demonstrated that one of the two fractions that could be prepared, chromatographically, from ceruloplasmin of a patient with Wilson's disease had a greater negative charge at pH 5.5 (but not at pH 8.6) than the same fraction from ceruloplasmin pooled from ten normal adults. This suggested that the abnormal fraction possessed a smaller number of histidine residues than the normal. Neifakh et al.[34] and Needleman et al.[35] prepared peptide maps by electrophoresis and chromatography of tryptic digests of ceruloplasmin. In the former study the peptide maps from both patients with Wilson's disease differed from the normal (and from each other), but in neither was there any net charge difference from the normal. In the latter study, the ceruloplasmin from one patient with Wilson's disease appeared to have two more positive charges than the protein from a normal donor. Interpretation of these results is complicated by the existence of a number of apparently normal polymorphisms of ceruloplasmin.[35a]

Neifakh et al.[34] also demonstrated a 50 per cent reduction in the specific oxidase activity of the ceruloplasmin isolated from the patients with Wilson's disease. Consistent with this result, Gollan[36] and Gibbs and Walshe[31] found that ceruloplasmin's specific oxidase activity, based on an immunochemical assay of the protein, was lower than normal in roughly half of the sera from patients with Wilson's disease, suggesting that the protein from the latter was less active as an oxidase but equally reactive immunochemically (perhaps as an apoprotein) than the normal protein.

If these limited and somewhat contradictory observations can be confirmed and reconciled they might account for the protein's deficiency: Although the intravascular survival of intravenously infused *normal* ceruloplasmin is no different in patients with Wilson's disease from that in control subjects,[26] we do not know whether ceruloplasmin of *abnormal* amino acid composition would have an abnormally short survival. If it did (and *normal* ceruloplasmin freed of its normal complement of sialic acid has a drastically shortened survival[29]), deficiency of ceruloplasmin would presumably result, unless the rate of synthesis of the protein were proportionately increased. It is also conceivable—and relevant to the pathogenesis of Wilson's disease (Chapter 4)—that the copper of an abnormally structured ceruloplasmin might not be excreted to the same degree as that of the normal protein.

2. *Decreased rate of synthesis.* Deficiency of ceruloplasmin would also occur if the rate of synthesis of the protein were abnormally low. Three sets of data give considerable support to this concept. First, Gaitskhoki et al.[37] found this to be true in in vitro studies comparing rates of ceruloplasmin synthesis in livers from patients with Wilson's disease and control subjects. They concluded tentatively that there was a decreased amount of translatable messenger RNA for ceruloplasmin in the patients' livers. Investigators from the same laboratory subsequently demonstrated that five discrete steps in the in vitro synthesis of the protein were impaired in patients' livers.[38]

Second, when frozen liver biopsy specimens were treated with fluorescein-conjugated anticeruloplasmin, no fluorescence was seen in the preparations made from patients with Wilson's disease, whereas fluorescence was visible in preparations from control subjects.[39] (The persuasiveness of these data, from which it would appear that there is no ceruloplasmin in Wilsonian hepatocytes, is lessened by the findings of Graul et al.,[40] who could find no difference between specimens of liver from patients with Wilson's disease and those from control subjects or from neonatal liver when they used an immunoperoxidase stain to identify ceruloplasmin in these samples. Graul et al. concluded that the deficiency of serum ceruloplasmin in Wilson's disease is caused either by defective copper incorporation into apoceruloplasmin or defective transport of ceruloplasmin from hepatocytes into serum.)

Third, the physiologic half-life of normal ceruloplasmin infused into patients with Wilson's disease does not differ from that injected into control subjects, suggesting (although with the caveat discussed above) that the deficiency of ceruloplasmin in Wilson's disease cannot be accounted for by an increased rate of catabolism of the protein.[26]

3. *Inhibition of synthesis.* Finally, it is possible that deficiency of ceruloplasmin may be a result of the persistence of the excessive amounts of copper present in all neonatal livers. Indeed, the normal (as well as the Wilsonian) infant—with both an elevated hepatic copper concentration *and* a reduced serum concentration of ceruloplasmin—may represent, in vivo, the in vitro finding that the combination of copper and apoceruloplasmin to form the holoprotein is markedly inhibited by an excess of copper.[5, 41, 42] Such a hypothesis would leave unexplained the invariable association of the normal (or elevated) concentrations of ceruloplasmin and the enormous concentrations of hepatic copper seen in primary biliary cirrhosis and Indian childhood cirrhosis.[43] The hypothesis is also difficult to reconcile with the presence of hypoceruloplasminemia and a normal or only slightly elevated hepatic copper concentration in about 20 per cent of the heterozygous carriers of one WD gene (see Chapter 4).

ANALYTIC METHODS

Ceruloplasmin can be quantitatively determined by (1) its enzymatic reaction with a variety of substrates,[44–50] (2) immunodiffusion,[51] (3) immunoelectrophoresis,[52] (4) nephelometry of an immune precipitate[53] or (5) electron paramagnetic resonance.[54]

REFERENCES

1. Holmberg, C. G., and Laurell, C.-B.: Investigations in serum copper. I. Nature of serum copper and its relation to the iron-binding protein in human serum. Acta Chem. Scand. *1*:944–950, 1947.
2. Holmberg, C. G., and Laurell, C.-B.: Investigations in serum copper. II. Isolation of the copper containing protein, and a description of some of its properties. Acta Chem. Scand. *2*:550–556, 1948.
3. Holmberg, C. G., and Laurell, C.-B.: Investigations in serum copper. III. Ceruloplasmin as an enzyme. Acta Chem. Scand. *5*:476–480, 1951.
4. Holmberg, C. G., and Laurell, C.-B.: Investigations in serum copper. IV. Effect of different anions on the enzymatic activity of ceruloplasmin. Acta Chem. Scand. *5*:921–930, 1951.
5. Scheinberg, I. H., Cook, C. D., and Murphy, J. A.: The concentration of copper and ceruloplasmin in maternal and infant plasma at delivery. J. Clin. Invest. *33*:963, 1954.
6. Danks, D. M.: Copper deficiency in humans. *In* Biological Roles of Copper. Ciba Foundation Symposium 79, Excerpta Medica, Amsterdam, 1980, pp. 209–225.
7. Lahey, M. E., Behar, M., Viteri, F., and Scrimshaw, N. S.: Values for copper, iron and iron-binding capacity in the serum in kwashiorkor. Pediatrics *22*:72–79, 1958.
8. Graham, G., and Cordano, A.: Copper deficiency in human subjects. *In* Trace Elements in Human Health and Disease. Ed. by Prasad, A. S. Academic Press, New York, 1976, pp. 363–372.
9. Markowitz, H., Gubler, C. J., Mahoney, J. P., Cartwright, G. E., and Wintrobe, M. M.: Studies on copper metabolism. XIV. Copper, ceruloplasmin and oxidase activity in sera of normal human subjects, pregnant women, and patients with infection, hepatolenticular degeneration and the nephrotic syndrome. J. Clin. Invest. *34*:1498–1508, 1955.
10. Sternlieb, I., and Janowitz, H. D.: Absorption of copper in malabsorption syndromes. J. Clin. Invest. *43*:1049–1055, 1964.
11. Cartwright, G. E.: The relationship of copper, cobalt and other trace elements to hemopoiesis. Amer. J. Clin. Nutr. *3*:11–19, 1955.
12. Butterworth, C. E., Jr., Gubler, C. J., Cartwright, G. E., and Wintrobe, M. M.: Studies on copper metabolism. XXVI. Plasma copper in patients with tropical sprue. Proc. Soc. Exptl. Biol. Med. *98*:594–597, 1958.
13. al-Rashid, R. A., and Spangler, J.: Neonatal copper deficiency. N. Engl. J. Med. *285*:841–843, 1971.
14. Cordano, A.: Copper deficiency in clinical medicine. *In* Zinc and Copper in Clinical Medicine. Ed. by Hambidge, K. M., and Nichols, B. L., Jr. Spectrum Publications, New York, 1978, pp. 119–126.
15. Walshe, J. M., and Briggs, J.: Caeruloplasmin in liver disease. A diagnostic pitfall. Lancet *II*:263–265, 1962.

15a. Morell, A. G., van den Hamer, C. J. A., and Scheinberg, I. H.: Physical and chemical studies on ceruloplasmin. VI. Preparation of human ceruloplasmin crystals. J. Biol. Chem. *244*:3494–3496, 1969.

15b. Magdoff-Fairchild, B., Lovell, F. M., and Low, B.: An x-ray crystallographic study of ceruloplasmin. Determination of molecular weight. J. Biol. Chem. *244*:3497–3499, 1969.

16. Rydén, L., and Björk, I.: Reinvestigation of some physicochemical and chemical properties of human ceruloplasmin (ferroxidase). Biochemistry *15*:3411–3417, 1976.
17. Dwulet, F. E., and Putman, F. W.: Complete amino acid sequence of a 50,000-dalton fragment of human ceruloplasmin. Proc. Natl. Acad. Sci. U.S.A. *78*:790–794, 1981.
18. Scheinberg, I. H., and Morell, A. G.: Ceruloplasmin. *In* Inorganic Biochemistry, Vol. 1. Ed. by Eichhorn, G. L. Elsevier, Amsterdam, 1973, pp. 306–319.
19. Noyer, M., Dwulet, F. E., Hao, Y. L., and Putnam, F. W.: Purification and characterization of undegraded human ceruloplasmin. Anal. Biochem. *102*:450–458, 1980.
20. Kingston, I. B., Kingston, B. L., and Putnam, F. W.: Primary structure of a histidine-rich proteolytic fragment of human ceruloplasmin. J. Biol. Chem. *255*:2886–2896, 1980.
21. Scheinberg, I. H.: Ceruloplasmin: A review. *In* Biochemistry of Copper. Ed. by Peisach, J., and Aisen, P. Academic Press, New York, 1966, pp. 513–524.
22. Frieden, E.: Caeruloplasmin: a multi-functional metalloprotein of vertebrate plasma. *In* Biological Roles of Copper. Ciba Foundation Symposium 79, Excerpta Medica, Amsterdam, 1980, pp. 93–124.
23. Feldman, S. L., Hunter, J. S. V., Zgirski, A., Chidambaram, M. V., and Frieden, E.: Comparison of the catalytic oxidation of cysteine and o-dianisidine by cupric ion and ceruloplasmin. J. Inorgan. Chem., 1982.
24. Morell, A. G., Aisen, P., and Scheinberg, I. H.: Is ceruloplasmin an ascorbic acid oxidase? J. Biol. Chem. *237*:3455–3457, 1962.
25. Yamashita, K., Liang, C. J., Funakoshi, S., and Kobata, A.: Structural studies of asparagine-linked sugar chains of human ceruloplasmin. J. Biol. Chem. *256*:1283–1289, 1981.
26. Sternlieb, I., Morell, A. G., Tucker, W. D., Greene, M. W., and Scheinberg, I. H.: The incorporation of copper into ceruloplasmin *in vivo*: studies with copper^{64} and copper^{67}. J. Clin. Invest. *40*:1834–1840, 1961.
27. Gitlin, D., and Janeway, C. A.: Genetic alterations in plasma proteins of man. *In* The Plasma Proteins, Vol. 2. Ed. by Putman, F. W. Academic Press, New York, 1960, pp. 407–451.

28. Campbell, C. H., Brown, R., and Linder, M. C.: Circulating ceruloplasmin is an important source of copper for normal and malignant cells. Biochim. Biophys. Acta *678*:27–38, 1981.
29. van den Hamer, C. J. A., Morell, A. G., and Scheinberg, I. H.: Physical and chemical studies on ceruloplasmin. IX. The role of galactosyl residues in the clearance of ceruloplasmin from the circulation. J. Biol. Chem. *245*:4397–4402, 1970.
30. Sternlieb, I., and Scheinberg, I. H.: Ceruloplasmin in health and disease. Ann. N.Y. Acad. Sci. *94*:71–76, 1961.
31. Gibbs, K., and Walshe, J. M.: A study of the caeruloplasmin concentrations found in 75 patients with Wilson's disease, their kinships and various control groups. Quart. J. Med. *48*:447–463, 1979.
32. Edwards, C. Q., Williams, D. M., and Cartwright, G. E.: Hereditary hypoceruloplasminemia. Clin. Genet. *15*:311–316, 1979.
32a. Sternlieb, I., and Scheinberg, I. H.: Chronic hepatitis as a first manifestation of Wilson's disease. Ann. Int. Med. *76*:59–64, 1972.
33. Hirschman, S. Z., Morell, A. G., and Scheinberg, I. H.: The heterogeneity of the copper-containing protein of human plasma ceruloplasmin. Ann. N.Y. Acad. Sci. *94*:960–969, 1961.
34. Neifakh, S. A., Vasiletz, I. M., and Shavlovsky, M. M.: Molecular pathology of ceruloplasmin. Biochem. Genet. *6*:231–238, 1972.
35. Needleman, S. B., Sahgal, V., and Boshes, B.: Studies on the biochemical characterization of human ceruloplasmin. Experientia *26*:495–496, 1970.
35a. Mohrenweiser, H. W., and Decker, R. S.: Identification of several electrophoretic variants of human ceruloplasmin including $Cp^{Michigan}$, a new polymorphism. Hum. Hered. *32*:369–373, 1982.
36. Gollan, J. L., Stocks, J., Dormany, T. L., and Sherlock, S.: Reduced oxidase activity in the ceruloplasmin of two families with Wilson's disease. J. Clin. Pathol. *30*:81–83, 1977.
37. Gaitskhoki, V. S., Kisselev, O. I., Moshkov, K. A., Puchkova, L. V., Shavlovski, M. M., Shulman, V. S., Vacharlovski, V. G., and Neifakh, S. A.: On the defect of synthesis ceruloplasmin in the liver polyribosomes in Wilson's disease. Biochem. Genet. *13*:533–550, 1975.
38. Neifakh, S. A., Vakharlovsky, V. G., Gaitskhoki, V. S., Monakhov, N. K., Puchkova, L. V., and Shvartsman, A. L.: Expression of the gene of ceruloplasmin in Konovalov-Wilson's disease. Vestn. Akad. Med. Nauk. USSR. *1*:53–63, 1982.
39. Shaposhnikov, A. M., Zubzitski, Y. N., and Shulman, V. S.: Identification of ceruloplasmin in human liver cells by fluorescent antibodies and absence of this protein in Wilson's disease. Experientia *25*:424–426, 1969.
40. Graul, R. S., Epstein, O., Sherlock, S., and Scheuer, P. J.: Immunocytochemical identification of caeruloplasmin in hepatocytes of patients with Wilson's disease. Liver *2*:207–211, 1982.
41. Morell, A. G., and Scheinberg, I. H.: Preparation of an apoprotein from ceruloplasmin by reversible dissociation of copper. Science *127*:588–590, 1958.
42. Bruckmann, G., and Zondek, S. G.: Iron, copper and manganese in human organs at various stages. Biochem. J. *33*:1845–1857, 1939.
43. Goldfischer, S., Popper, H., and Sternlieb, I.: The significance of variations in the distribution of copper in liver disease. Amer. J. Pathol. *99*:715–730, 1980.
44. Ravin, H. A.: An improved colorimetric enzymatic assay for ceruloplasmin. J. Lab. Clin. Med. *58*:161–168, 1961.
45. O'Reilly, S.: A modified oxidase assay for low concentrations of ceruloplasmin in serum and other biological fluids. Neurology *12*:400–466, 1962.
46. Johnson, D. A., Osaki, S., and Frieden, E.: A micromethod for the determination of ferroxidase (ceruloplasmin) in human serums. Clin. Chem. *13*:142–150, 1967.
47. Morell, A. G., Windsor, J., Sternlieb, I., and Scheinberg, I. H.: Measurement of the concentrations of ceruloplasmin in serum by determination of its oxidase activity. *In* Laboratory Diagnosis of Liver Diseases. Ed. by Sunderman, F. W., and Sunderman, F. W., Jr. Warren H. Green, St. Louis, 1968, pp. 193–195.
48. Jérôme, H. and Girault, M.: Dosage de la céruloplasmine; normalisation des résultats. Anal. Biol. Chem. *27*:371–385, 1969.
49. Sunderman, F. W., Jr., and Nomoto, S.: Measurement of human serum ceruloplasmin by its p-phenylenediamine oxidase activity. Clin. Chem. *16*:903–910, 1970.
50. Schosinksky, K. H., Lehmann, H. P., and Beeler, M. F.: Automated determination of serum ceruloplasmin activity with o-dianisidine dihydrochloride as substrate. Clin. Chem. *21*:757–759, 1975.
51. Sandor, G., Martin, L., Mattern, P., Orely, C., Sureau, B., Berrod, J., and Martin, R.: Immunserums correspondent à des composants protéidiques individuels du serum humain. Leur application à l'immunochimie quantitative par la méthode de diffusion radiale. II. Résultats obtenus sur une grande échelle en pathologie humaine. Ann. Inst. Pasteur *113*:569–590, 1967.
52. Laurell, C.-B.: Quantitative estimation of protein by electrophoresis in agarose containing antibodies. Anal. Biochem. *15*:45–52, 1966.
53. Pesce, M. A., and Bodourian, S. H.: Nephelometric measurement of ceruloplasmin with a centrifugal analyzer. Clin. Chem. *28*:516–519, 1982.
54. Pocklington, T., and Foster, M. A.: Electron spin resonance of caeruloplasmin and iron transferrin in blood in patients with various malignant diseases. Brit. J. Cancer *36*:369–374, 1977.
55. Sass-Kortsak, A., and Bearn, A. G.: Hereditary disorders of copper metabolism. *In* The Metabolic Basis of Inherited Disease, 4th ed. Ed. by Stanbury, J. B., Wyngaarden, J. B., and Fredrickson, D. S. McGraw-Hill, New York, 1978, pp. 1098–1126.

CHAPTER 4

PATHOGENESIS

In Wilson's disease, the primary pathogenetic mechanism is the inherited metabolic defect that is always associated with the gradual and progressive accumulation of copper in the liver.[1,2] The first definite chemical abnormality caused by this defect is a copper concentration of the order of 1000 mcg/g dry liver—more than 20 times normal—by three or four years of age (see Fig. 5–2). Although histopathologic changes due to this excess copper are apparent in the liver even earlier in life, clinically apparent hepatic dysfunction is almost never seen before the age of five or six years, and may not be manifest for decades. Extrahepatic copper toxicity occurs when the liver's burden of copper becomes so great that the metal is released into the blood stream, whence it can diffuse into the brain and other organs—a process that understandably *decreases* the copper content of the liver as the concentration of the metal in other tissues rises (Table 4–1 and Fig. 4–1). The secondary pathogenetic events are those that result in copper toxicity to these systems.

PRIMARY PATHOGENESIS: ACCUMULATION OF EXCESS COPPER

Ceruloplasmin and the Pathogenesis of Wilson's Disease

Although it is certain, as documented later in this chapter and in Chapter 3, that ceruloplasmin is closely related to the primary genetic defect in Wilson's disease, it is not clear whether a genetic abnormality in the synthesis of this protein causes copper to accumulate to excess. Hypotheses of such a cause-and-effect relationship are of two types. The first postulates synthesis of too little of the normal protein; the second postulates synthesis of a structurally and functionally abnormal ceruloplasmin.

Since about 0.5 mg of copper is required normally for the amount of

TABLE 4–1. Concentration of Copper in Tissues of Authors' Patients with Wilson's Disease and Control Subjects Obtained at Autopsy (mcg/g dry tissue)

Tissue	Untreated				Partially Treated				Treated				Normal	
	No. of Patients	Copper Concentration			No. of Patients	Copper Concentration			No. of Patients	Copper Concentration			Copper Concentration	
		Range	*Mean**	*S.D.*		*Range*	*Mean*	*S.D.*		*Range*	*Mean*	*S.D.*	*Range*	*Mean*
Liver	21	128–2217	926 (541)	±599	5	223–1605	895	±634	11	18–829	291	±263	9–47	26
Heart	3	79–298	157 (13)	—	2	22, 137	80	—	7	14–84	35	± 26	10–23	17
Kidney	11	12–1246	556 (83)	±407	3	66–2045	1128	—	9	9–40	19	± 12	5–36	15
Spleen	5	1–100	45 (7)	± 38	1	7	—	—	3	6–42	21	—	3–16	7
Brain														
Cerebral cortex gray	12	93–297	195 (275)	± 73	4	70–210	123	± 62	9	25–335	169	±112	20–33	26
White matter	6	33–297	141 (149)	±121	1	107	—	—	5	77–234	140	± 73	10–16	13
Cerebellum	—	—	(271)	—	1	151	—	—	3	76–421	209	—	6–18	14
Basal ganglion	3	58–221	141 (225)	—	2	66,106	86	—	3	58–226	124	—	10–43	31
Caudate nucleus	3	62–188	121 (231)	—	2	171,191	181	—	1	236	—	—	20–43	29
Thalamus	1	179	(436)	—	1	243	—	—	1	226	—	—	13–19	16
Globus pallidus	—	—	(226)	—	—	—	—	—	—	—	—	—	10–43	30
Putamen	4	120–224	175 (378)	± 50	1	210	—	—	5	85–252	174	± 63	23–43	33
Medulla	3	60–280	190 (237)	—	1	231	—	—	2	208,258	233	—		
Substantia nigra	—	—	—	—	—	—	—	—	1	196	—	—	44–77	60
Pons	2	44,140	92	—	1	140	—	—	2	36,122	79	—	4–10	7
Spinal cord	1	90	—	—	—	—	—	—	3	12,142	59	—	3–16	9
Cornea	—	—	—	—	1	456	—	—	1	15	—	—		

*Numbers in parentheses represent the mean of analyses by nine groups of investigators culled from the literature.

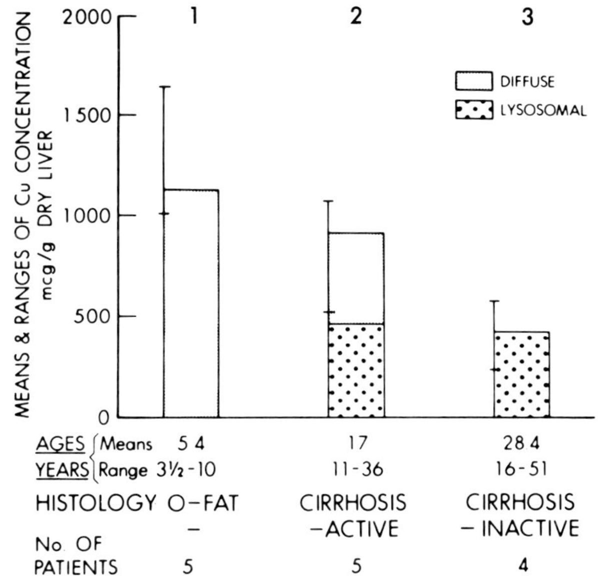

Figure 4–1. Mean values and ranges of hepatic copper concentrations in patients with Wilson's disease grouped according to age and stage of the disease. 1. Young, asymptomatic patients with minimal histologic abnormalities; 2. adolescents and young adults with active liver disease; and 3. adults with neurologic Wilson's disease and inactive cirrhosis. The height of the bar graphs indicates the concentration of copper in each group. There is a striking decrease with advancing age and progression of the disease, and the intracellular distribution of copper changes from its diffuse cytoplasmic distribution in the hepatocytes of the young patients to its lysosomal concentration in the hepatocytes of the patient with advanced disease.

ceruloplasmin synthesized and catabolized daily,[3] and since ceruloplasmin-copper is probably excreted when the protein is catabolized,[4, 5] deficient synthesis of the protein could easily result in the retention of an amount of copper sufficient to produce the excess accumulations seen in these patients. And the copper of a structurally abnormal ceruloplasmin might not be excreted normally.

From the discussion of the evidence relevant to both hypotheses in Chapter 3, it is clear that neither has been proven true. Even if either were established, however, it would be difficult to equate it to the inherited defect because of two kinds of individuals: patients with Wilson's disease who exhibit normal concentrations of ceruloplasmin, sometimes for years; and clinically unaffected heterozygous carriers of one WD gene with deficiency (occasionally marked) of ceruloplasmin (see Chapter 3).

Therefore, theories that have been advanced—including one of ours[6]—causally relating abnormalities of ceruloplasmin to the pathogenesis of Wilson's disease appear untenable. Despite this, it seems quite possible that a pathogenetic role for ceruloplasmin in Wilson's disease will eventually be discovered. Perhaps the most compelling reason for such a belief is the fact that except for the excessive accumulations of tissue copper that cause Wilson's disease, no abnormality has been shown to be associated with deficiency of ceruloplasmin, even in those patients with

Wilson's disease who possess no detectable quantity of the protein in the circulation. What is ceruloplasmin doing physiologically, we must ask, if it is not preventing the development of Wilson's disease?

Excessive Absorption of Copper and Wilson's Disease

Normally less than half of the dietary copper is absorbed from the gastrointestinal tract.[7–10] A number of investigations have been made to determine whether the inherited defect in Wilson's disease leads to greater than normal absorption of the metal or to less than normal excretion, either situation resulting in excessive copper accumulation.[11–13] Balance studies cannot discriminate between these two causes. But measurements of the maximal concentration of copper attained in the blood after the ingestion of a radiocopper salt—numbers that may reasonably be assumed to be proportional to the extent of absorption—have not been consistently different in patients with Wilson's disease from those in control subjects.[14, 15]

Biliary Excretion of Copper and Wilson's Disease

There is evidence from four laboratories that biliary excretion of copper is impaired in patients with Wilson's disease.[16–19] Since urinary excretion of copper is negligible, and since van Berge Henegouwen et al.[20] have shown by careful perfusion studies that the normal adult excretes about 50 per cent of ingested (and therefore almost all of the absorbed) copper in the bile, even a small reduction in biliary excretion of copper could readily account for these patients' positive balances.

In one study designed to investigate the abnormality in biliary excretion of copper in Wilson's disease, radiocopper was administered to two women—one with Wilson's disease—18 hours before cholecystectomy.[19] At surgery, specimens were taken to permit determinations of the specific activities and total concentrations of copper in bile and subcellular fractions of liver. In the patient with Wilson's disease the lysosomal and biliary concentrations of total copper were, respectively, much greater and much lower than in the control subject. Moreover, in the woman with Wilson's disease, there was near equality of the specific activity of lysosomal and biliary copper, indicating that the source of the latter was lysosomal. These three observations, though shedding no light on its mechanism, suggest that the site of the excretory defect is localized to lysosomes (Table 4–2).

One Defect Impairing Ceruloplasmin Synthesis and Biliary Copper Excretion

In 1965 Sass-Kortsak hypothesized that "the basic defect in Wilson's disease probably concerns a mechanism by which copper is made available,

TABLE 4–2. Copper and Radiocopper Concentrations in Liver Homogenates, Subcellular Fractions, Bile and Serum of a Control Subject and a Patient with Wilson's Disease[19]

	TOTAL COPPER (μg/g* or ml)		^{64}COPPER (ng/g* or ml)		SPECIFIC ACTIVITY (^{64} CU/TOTAL COPPER)	
	Control	*W.D.*	*Control*	*W.D.*	*Control*	*W.D.*
Liver homogenate	7.10	62.20	31.3	100.0	4.42	1.610
Nuclear fraction	0.41	6.80	0.60	1.8	1.46	0.265
Mitochondrial fraction	0.60	9.40	0.92	1.5	1.53	0.160
Lysosomal fraction	0.37	15.90	0.84	1.3	2.27	0.082
Microsomal fraction	0.68	3.30	1.33	2.1	1.95	0.637
Cytosol	5.78	21.10	26.80	83.2	4.64	3.950
Common duct bile	10.47	1.73	43.3	0.15	4.13	0.087
Serum	1.19	0.77	3.2	1.7	2.70	2.20

*Wet weight of liver.

From Sternlieb, I., et al. Gastroenterology *64*:99–105, 1973. With permission of the publisher. Copyright 1973 by the American Gastroenterological Association.

or presented in a suitably activated form, both for excretion via the bile and for incorporation into ceruloplasmin."[7] Epstein and Sherlock have linked ceruloplasmin synthesis and biliary copper excretion in a more detailed hypothesis suggesting that "mutation of a single gene causes the impairment of both caeruloplasmin synthesis and biliary copper excretion" in Wilson's disease.[21] They believe that "the disease results from failure to switch from the positive copper balance of the fetus to the normal copper balance of the child." This maladaptation, they hypothesize, accounts for the etiologic "relentless accumulation of copper in the liver after birth." Such a concept of a controller gene that *directly* impairs *both* ceruloplasmin synthesis and biliary copper excretion seems to us incompatible with the following clinical observations.

Normal concentrations of ceruloplasmin are present in about 5 per cent of patients with Wilson's disease, presumably because in some patients synthesis can be induced by such factors as estrogens or inflammation. Epstein and Sherlock's hypothesis is, therefore, compatible with a dissociation of ceruloplasmin synthesis and biliary copper excretion as a result of which a patient with Wilson's disease may exhibit a *normal* ceruloplasmin concentration and a *diminished* biliary excretion of copper. However, except for the neonatal state; Menkes' disease; a very rare form of non-Wilsonian, inherited, hypoceruloplasminemia[22]; the nephrotic syndrome; protein-losing gastroenteropathy; kwashiorkor; marasmus; or severe copper-deficiency, we are unaware of any genetic, physiologic, pharmacologic, or pathologic factor that can induce *deficiency* of ceruloplasmin in an individual who does not possess at least one WD gene. Consequently, we assume that the deficiency of ceruloplasmin seen in about 20 per cent of healthy heterozygous carriers of one WD gene must be caused by that gene.[2] In three such heterozygotes (M7, R3 and M8) we have observed marked deficiency of ceruloplasmin without excessive concentrations of hepatic copper and therefore, we assume, without significant impairment of biliary copper excretion (Table 4–3). Walshe has agreed implicitly with our conclusion that these data cannot be reconciled with a gene that regulates both ceruloplasmin synthesis and biliary excretion of copper.[23]

TABLE 4–3. Ceruloplasmin, Hepatic Copper Concentrations and Hepatic Histology in Patients with Wilson's Disease, Heterozygotes, and Normal Subjects

SUBJECTS AND AGE	CERULOPLASMIN (mg/dl)	HEPATIC COPPER (mcg/g/ dry wt.)	HISTOLOGY
M7, 51 yr., patient's mother	1.9; <1*	23.6; 54.8†	Normal
R3, 9 yr., patient's son	12	136	Normal
M8, 27 yr., patient's brother	<1; 1.9‡	257	Normal
Heterozygotes[2]	1–50	39–213	Normal
Wilson's disease[2]	<1–19.5	>250	Abnormal
Normal subjects[2]	18.5–65.9	20–45	Normal

*Five years between the first ceruloplasmin analysis, at age 51, and the second.
†Four months between hepatic biopsies at age 51.
‡16 years between the first ceruloplasmin analysis, at age 27, and the second.

SECONDARY PATHOGENETIC MECHANISMS

Whatever is awry in Wilson's disease, copper accumulates far in excess of the metabolic requirements for this metal. The normal state of copper in vivo—in which virtually all of the metal is present as a tightly bound prosthetic element of about a dozen physiologic copper-proteins—is drastically altered. Excess copper combines with cellular or molecular sulfhydryl, carboxyl, or amino groups, where it does not belong, interfering with the structure or function of molecules. The following examples of what abnormal effects copper can produce are not all derived from observations made in humans or on liver. Copper can (1) cause profound morphologic changes in mitochondria[24, 25] and peroxisomes[25, 26] in the hepatocytes of patients with Wilson's disease; (2) affect the integrity of the plasma membrane[27, 27a]; (3) degrade microtubules[28] or prevent the polymerization of tubulin[29]; (4) promote labilization of lysosomal membranes, with consequent leakage of copper (as well as enzymes) into the cytosol, where both may cause further harm[30–32]; (5) oxidize reduced glutathione, reducing the cell's reserves of this essential metabolite[33]; and (6) cause cross-linking and destabilization of nuclear DNA.[34] Other effects of copper on cellular elements of the liver are presented in Table 4–4.

TABLE 4–4. Experimental Effects of Added Copper on Cellular Elements of Liver

CELLULAR PREPARATIONS, ELEMENTS AND ENZYMES	SPECIES	EFFECT	REFERENCES
Glutathione, reduced	Rat	Diminution	33
Homogenate	Rat	Glycogen content increased; phospholipids decreased; acid phosphatase increased	76
Isolated hepatocytes	Rat	Viability decreased	33
Mitochondria	Rat	Swelling; rearranged cristae	27,30
	Rat	Respiration inhibited; oxidative phosphorylation uncoupled	76a
Polysomes	Rat	Diminution and dissociation	66
	Rabbit	Diminution of heavy polysomes	78
Acid phosphatase (microsomal, lysosomal, cytosolic)	Rat	Enzyme activity increased	30
N-Acetyl-β-D-glucosaminidase (lysosomal)	Rat	Enzyme activity increased	30
Aniline hydroxylase (microsomal)	Rat	Enzyme activity decreased	79
Dopa decarboxylase	Rat	Enzyme activity decreased	33a
Epoxide hydrase (microsomal)	Rat	Enzyme activity decreased	80
β-Glucuronidase (lysosomal)	Rat	Enzyme activity increased	30
Glutathione reductase	Rat	Enzyme activity decreased	81
Lactate dehydrogenase	Rat	Enzyme activity decreased	33a
Malate dehydrogenase	Mouse	Enzyme activity decreased	30
Monoamine oxidase	Rat	Enzyme activity decreased	33a
Succinate dehydrogenase	Rat	Enzyme activity decreased	33a

More speculatively, copper, by its affinity for sulfhydryl groups, may promote the polymerization of copper-thionein[35] and, by its effects on microtubules and tubulin, may inhibit the export of triglycerides or lipoproteins from hepatocytes, resulting, perhaps, in the steatosis characteristic of the early stages of Wilson's disease or in the formation of the Mallory bodies seen in patients with submassive hepatic necrosis. Studies on the inherited copper toxicosis of Bedlington terriers suggest that excess copper may stimulate fibrogenesis even in the absence of either cell necrosis or parenchymal collapse.[36]

Irrespective of whether the invariable hepatic pathology is accompanied by significant clinical liver disease, sooner or later copper is released from that organ. If this occurs suddenly, as a consequence of copper-induced hepatic necrosis, large amounts of copper ions rapidly enter the blood stream. Hemolytic anemia, commonly seen in this situation, is probably caused by an increased plasma concentration of free copper[37–39] that can reach levels capable of interfering, at least in vitro, with a number of erythrocytic functions (Table 4–5).[40–57] However, very few instances of hemolytic anemia have been reported in which the plasma concentrations of free, nonceruloplasmin copper approach the concentrations used in the in vitro studies.[57a]

TABLE 4–5. Experimental Effects of Copper on Components of Erythrocytes

COMPONENTS	EFFECT	REFERENCES
Enzymes and Cofactors		
Adenosine triphosphate (ATP)	Utilization diminished	40
Catalase	Diminished	41
δ-Aminolevulinic acid dehydratase	Inhibited	42
Glucose-6-phosphate dehydrogenase (G-6-PD)	Inhibited	38,43–46
	Unaffected	47
Glutathione	Diminished	38,41,46–48
	Unchanged	49
	Oxidized	45
Glutathione reductase	Inhibited	38,41,49a
Heme oxygenase	Stimulated	50
Hexokinase	Inhibited	44
Nicotinamide adenine dinucleotide, reduced (NADH)	Oxidation enhanced	45
	Oxidation unchanged	38
Phosphofructokinase	Inhibited	44
6-Phosphogluconate dehydrogenase	Inhibited	44
Phosphoglyceric kinase	Inhibited	44
Pyruvate kinase	Inhibited	44,47
Other Components		
Glycerol	Uptake impaired	51
Hemoglobin	Oxidized, denatured, forming methemoglobin and Heinz bodies	52–54
Membrane lipids	Peroxidized	39
Membrane protein	Increased cross-linking and rigidity	55–57

More often the egress of copper from the liver is gradual, and the toxic effects of its diffusion into the brain, kidney, eye and other organs appear insidiously over years or decades. During this latent period, which may also follow an episode of hepatic necrosis and hemolytic anemia, the activity of the copper-induced liver disease generally subsides. Even with an episode of severe hepatitis in the past, chemical tests of liver dysfunction are now little, if at all, affected despite the presence of regenerated nodules and scar tissue. Individual hepatocytes may appear completely normal, except for prominent copper-laden lysosomal granules: The capacity of lysosomes to sequester copper late in the disease apparently protects the hepatocyte from further toxic effects.[25, 58]

The pathologic changes in the brain in Wilson's disease are always associated with marked elevations of tissue copper content, although clinical data relating these directly to the effects of copper on the brain are scarce. Dopamine beta hydroxylase has been found to be reduced in one patient,[58a] and measurements of cerebrospinal fluid components have been interpreted as indicating damage to dopaminergic and serotonergic neurones.[58b] Experimentally (Table 4–6), copper has been shown to inhibit oxidation in isolated brain mitochondria[59]; to impair mitochondrial monoamine oxidase,[59a] Na^+, K^+-ATPase,[60–62] adenylate cyclase and phosphodiesterase activities[63]; and to decrease the accumulation of monoamines in synaptosomes,[64] possibly interfering with neurotransmission. Injections of copper into the ventricles of cats produces spongy degeneration.[65]

We do not know how, or whether, these experimental findings are related to the pathologic glial and neuronal lesions or functional changes seen in patients with Wilson's disease. But, although some of the histo-

TABLE 4–6. Experimental Effects of Added Copper on Cellular Elements and Compounds of the Central Nervous System

Preparations, Enzymes and Catecholamines	Species	Effect	References
Homogenate	Rat	Respiration inhibited	61,65a
Polysomes	Rat	Diminished	66
Adenylate cyclase (membrane)	Rat	Enzyme activity inhibited	63,67
Na^+,K^+–Adenosinetriphosphatase (ATPase) (microsomal)	Chicken, pigeon, rat	Enzyme inactivated	61,62,68–70,70a
	Beef	Enzyme activity inhibited	71
Na^+,K^+–ATPase (synaptosomal)	Rat	Enzyme activity inhibited	60
N-Methyltransferase	Rabbit	Enzyme activity inhibited	72
Monoamine oxidase	Rat	Enzyme activity inhibited	33a,59a
Phosphodiesterase	Rat	Enzyme activity inhibited	73
Dopamine (synaptosomal)	Rat	Uptake inhibited	64
5-Hydroxyindoleacetic acid	Rat	Diminished	33a
6-Hydroxydopamine (synaptosomal)	In vitro	Autoxidation stimulated	74
5-Hydroxytryptamine (synaptosomal)	Rat	Uptake inhibited	64
Noradrenaline	Rat	Uptake inhibited	64

pathologic lesions of Wilson's disease—the presence of Alzheimer Types I and II glia, Opalski cells, and cavitation of the basal ganglia—resemble those seen in hepatic encephalopathy, we believe, for three reasons, that the histologic and physiologic pathology of the central nervous system is caused by copper toxicity and *not*, as some authors have suggested,[75] by the effects of portosystemic shunting. First, many patients with severe neurologic manifestations of Wilson's disease have no such shunting or even any significant hepatic dysfunction. Second, treatment for hepatic encephalopathy has virtually no effect in patients with Wilson's disease, whereas decoppering therapy with penicillamine is often dramatic. Third, in unpublished observations, Horoupian and we have observed—in those few patients who have come to autopsy following treatment with penicillamine that produced significant improvement in neurologic disturbances—that there were relatively few histopathologic changes and markedly diminished copper concentrations.

Both copper, in Wilson's disease, and ammonia, in hepatic-encephalopathy due to portosystemic shunting, may, however, alter brain function by damaging microtubules. That copper can do this to protozoan microtubules has been mentioned above[28]; portacaval anastomosis in rats can raise plasma-ammonia levels and produce Alzheimer I glia, apparently by an effect on microtubules.[75a] If microtubules are essential to the physiology of neurones, it is possible that the remarkable reversibility of the neurologic manifestations so often seen in Wilson's disease is a consequence, in part, of the reversible nature of copper's damage to neuronal microtubules.

What little is known of the pathogenesis of Wilsonian lesions in the kidney, eye, pancreas, heart, integument and skeletal system is described in the chapters on those structures.

REFERENCES

1. Cumings, J. N.: Heavy Metals and the Brain, Charles C Thomas, Springfield, Ill., 1959.
2. Sternlieb, I., and Scheinberg, I. H.: Prevention of Wilson's disease in asymptomatic patients. N. Engl. J. Med. *278*:352–359, 1968.
3. Sternlieb, I., Morell, A. G., Tucker, W. D., Greene, M. W., and Scheinberg, I. H.: The incorporation of copper into ceruloplasmin *in vivo*: studies with ^{64}copper and ^{67}copper. J. Clin. Invest. *40*:1834–1840, 1961.
4. Gregoriadis, G., Morell, A. G., Sternlieb, I., and Scheinberg, I. H.: Catabolism of desialylated ceruloplasmin in the liver. J. Biol. Chem. *245*:5833–5837, 1970.
5. Kressner, M., Sternlieb, I., Stockert, R. J., and Morell, A. G.: Origins of biliary copper. Gastroenterology *82*:1232, 1982.
6. Scheinberg, I. H., and Morell, A. G.: Exchange of ceruloplasmin copper with ionic Cu^{64} with reference to Wilson's disease. J. Clin. Invest. *36*:1193–1201, 1957.
7. Sass-Kortsak, A.: Copper metabolism. Adv. Clin. Chem. *8*:1–67, 1965.
8. Sternlieb, I.: Gastrointestinal copper absorption. Gastroenterology *52*:1038–1041, 1967.
9. Spencer, H., Asmussen, C. R., Holtzman, R. B., and Kramer, L.: Metabolic balances of cadmium, copper, manganese, and zinc in man. Amer. J. Clin. Nutr. *32*:1867–1875, 1979.
10. Bremner, I.: Absorption, transport and distribution of copper. *In* Biological Roles of Copper. Ciba Foundation Symposium 79, Excerpta Medica, Amsterdam, 1980, pp. 23–48.
11. Tu, J.-B., Cooper, W. C., Blackwell, R. Q., and Hou, T. Y.: Asymptomatic Wilson's disease. Acta Paed. Sinica *3*:154–160, 1962.
12. Goldstein, N. P., Randall, R. V., Gross, J. B., and McGuckin, W. F.: Copper balance studies in Wilson's disease: observations on the effect of penicillamine, carbacrylamine resins, and potassium sulfide. Arch. Neurol. *12*:456–462, 1965.
13. Strickland, G. T., Blackwell, R. Q., and Watten, R. H.: Metabolic studies in Wilson's disease. Evaluation of efficacy of chelation therapy in respect to copper balance. Amer. J. Med. *51*:31–40, 1971.

14. Sternlieb, I., Morell, A. G., Bauer, C. D., Combes, B., DeBobes-Sternberg, S., and Scheinberg, I. H.: Detection of the heterozygous carrier of the Wilson's disease gene. J. Clin. Invest. *40*:707–715, 1961.
15. Sternlieb, I., and Scheinberg, I. H.: Radiocopper in diagnosing liver disease. Sem. Nucl. Med. *2*:176–188, 1972
16. O'Reilly, S., Weber, P. M., Oswald, M., and Shipley, L.: Abnormalities of the physiology of copper in Wilson's disease. III. The excretion of copper. Arch. Neurol. *25*:28–32, 1971.
17. Frommer, D. J.: Defective biliary excretion of copper in Wilson's disease. Gut *15*:125–129, 1974.
18. Gibbs, K., and Walshe, J. M.: Biliary excretion of copper in Wilson's disease. Lancet *II*:538–539, 1980.
19. Sternlieb, I., van den Hamer, C. J. A., Morell, A. G., Alpert, S., Gregoriadis, G., and Scheinberg, I. H.: Lysosomal defect of hepatic copper excretion in Wilson's disease (hepatolenticular degeneration). Gastroenterology *64*:99–105, 1973.
20. van Berge Henegouwen, G. P., Tangedahl, T. N., Hoffman, A. F., Northfield, T. C., LaRusso, N. F., and McCall, J. T.: Biliary secretion of copper in healthy man. Gastroenterology *72*:1228–1231, 1977.
21. Epstein, O., and Sherlock, S.: Is Wilson's disease caused by a controller gene mutation resulting in perpetuation of the fetal mode of copper metabolism into childhood? Lancet *I*:303–305, 1981.
22. Edwards, C. Q., Williams, D. M., and Cartwright, G. E.: Hereditary hypoceruloplasminemia. Clin. Gen. *15*:311–316, 1979.
23. Walshe, J. M.: Wilson's disease (hepatolenticular degeneration). *In* Handbook of Clinical Neurology. Ed. by Vinken, P. J., and Bruyn, G. W. Elsevier, Oxford, 1976, pp. 379–414.
24. Sternlieb, I.: Mitochondrial and fatty changes in hepatocytes of patients with Wilson's disease. Gastroenterology *5*:354–367, 1968.
25. Sternlieb, I.: Evolution of the hepatic lesion of Wilson's disease (hepatolenticular degeneration). *In* Progress in Liver Diseases, Vol. IV. Ed. by Popper, H., and Schaffner, F. Grune & Stratton, New York, 1972, pp. 511–525.
26. Sternlieb, I., and Quintana, N.: Abnormalities of human hepatocellular peroxisomes. Ann. N. Y. Acad. Sci. *386*:530–533, 1982.
27. Verity, M. A., and Gambell, J. K.: Studies of copper ion-induced mitochondrial swelling *in vitro*. Biochem. J. *108*:289–295, 1968.
27a. Kumar, K. S., Rowse, C., and Hochstein, P.: Copper-induced generation of superoxide in human red cell membranes. Biochem. Biophys. Res. Commun. *83*:587–592, 1978.
28. Roth, L. E., and Shigenaka, T.: Microtubules in the heliozoan axopodium. II. Rapid degradation by cupric and nickelous ions. J. Ultrastruct. Res. *31*:356–374, 1970.
29. Wallin, M., Larsson, H., and Edstrom, A.: Tubulin sulfhydryl groups and polymerization in vitro. Effects of di- and trivalent cations. Exp. Cell Res. *31*:356–374, 1970.
30. Verity, M. A., Gambell, J. K., Reith, A. R., and Brown, W. J.: Subcellular distribution and enzyme changes following subacute copper intoxication. Lab. Invest. *16*:580–590, 1967.
31. McNatt, E. N., Campbell, W. G., Jr., and Callahan, B. C.: Effects of dietary copper loading on livers of rats. I. Changes in subcellular acid phosphatases and detection of an additional acid p-nitrophenylphosphatase in the cellular supernatant during copper loading. Amer. J. Pathol. *64*:123–144, 1971.
32. Lindquist, R. R.: Studies on the pathogenesis of hepatolenticular degeneration. III. The effect of copper on rat liver lysosomes. Amer. J. Pathol. *53*:903–927, 1968.
33. Stacey, N. H., and Klassen, C. D.: Copper toxicity in isolated rat hepatocytes. Toxicol. Appl. Pharmacol. *58*:211–220, 1981.
33a. Lal, S., Papeschi, R., Duncan, R. J. S., and Soukes, T. L.: Effect of copper loading on various tissue enzymes and brain monoamines in the rat. Toxicol. Appl. Pharmacol. *28*:395–405, 1974.
34. Eichhorn, G. L., and Clark, P.: The unwinding and rewinding of DNA strands under the influence of copper (II) ions. Proc. Natl. Acad. Sci. U.S.A. *53*:586–593, 1965.
35. Morell, A. G., Shapiro, J. R., and Scheinberg, I. H.: Copper binding protein of human liver. *In* Wilson's Disease: Some Current Concepts. Ed. by Walshe, J. M., and Cumings, J. N. Blackwell, Oxford, 1961, pp. 36–42.
36. Twedt, D. C., Sternlieb, I., and Gilbertson, S.: Clinical, morphologic and chemical studies on copper toxicosis of Bedlington terriers. J. Amer. Vet. Med. Assoc. *175*:269–275, 1979.
37. Sherlock, S., McIntyre, N., Clink, H. M., Levi, A. J., and Cumings, J. N.: Hemolytic anemia in Wilson's disease. *In* Wilson's Disease. Birth Defects, Original Artricle Series, Vol. IV. Ed. by Bergsma, D., Scheinberg, I. H., and Sternlieb, I. The National Foundation—March of Dimes, New York, 1968, pp. 99–102.
38. Deiss, A., Lee, G. R., and Cartwright, G. E.: Hemolytic anemia in Wilson's disease. Ann. Int. Med. *73*:413–418, 1970.
39. Forman, S. J., Kumar, K. S., Redeker, A. G., and Hochstein, P.: Hemolytic anemia in Wilson's disease: clinical findings and biochemical mechanisms. Amer. J. Hematol. *9*:269–275, 1980.
40. Feig, S. A., Segel, G. B., Shohet, S. B., and Nathan, D. G.: Energy metabolism in human erythrocytes. II. Effects of glucose depletion. J. Clin. Invest. *51*:1547–1554, 1972.
41. Metz, E. N., and Sagone, A. L., Jr.: The effect of copper on the erythrocyte hexose monophosphate shunt pathway. J. Lab. Clin. Med. *80*:405–413, 1972.
42. Nelson, H. M., Hughes, M. A., and Meredith, P. A.: Zinc, copper and delta-aminolaevulinic acid dehydratase *in vitro* and *in vivo*. Toxicology *21*:261–266, 1981.

43. Passwell, J., Cohen, B. E., Ben Bassat, I., Ramot, B., Shchory, M., and Lavi, U.: Hemolysis in Wilson's disease. The role of glucose–6–phosphate dehydrogenase inhibition. Isr. J. Med. Sci. *6*:549–554, 1970.
44. Boulard, M., Blume, K.-G., and Beutler, E.: The effect of copper on red cell enzyme activities. J. Clin. Invest. *52*:459–461, 1972.
45. Fairbanks, V. F.: Copper sulfate induced hemolytic anemia. Arch. Int. Med. *120*:428–432, 1967.
46. Calabrese, E. J., Moore, G. S., and Ho, S.-C.: Low glucose–6–phosphate dehydrogenase (G–6–PD) activity in red blood cells and susceptibility to copper-induced oxidative damage. Environ. Res. *21*:366–372, 1980.
47. Willms, B., Blume, K. G., and Lohr, G. W.: Hämolytische Anämie bei Morbus Wilson (Hepatolentikuläre Degeneration). Klin. Wschr. *50*:995–1002, 1972.
48. Thompson, R. H., and Todd, J. R.: Role of pentose-phosphate pathway in a haemolytic crisis of chronic copper toxicity of sheep. Res. Vet. Sci. *20*:257–269, 1976.
49. Hiroshige, Y.: The effects of copper and copper o-phenanthroline complex on the intact human erythrocytes. Tohoku J. Exp. Med. *130*:385–402, 1980.
49a. Flikweert, J. P., Hoorn, R. K. J., and Staal, G. E. J.: The effect of copper on human erythrocyte glutathione reductase. Int. J. Biochem. *5*:649–653, 1974.
50. Maines, M. D., and Kappas, A.: Metals as regulators of heme metabolism. Science *198*:1215–1221, 1977.
51. Jacobs, M. H., and Corson, S. A.: The influence of minute traces of copper on certain hemolytic processes. Biol. Bull. *67*:325–326, 1934.
52. Winterbourn, C. C., and Carrell, R. W.: Oxidation of human haemoglobin by copper. Mechanism and suggested role of the thiol group of residue beta-93. Biochem. J. *165*:141–148, 1977.
53. Rifkind, J. M.: Copper and the autoxidation of hemoglobin. Biochemistry *13*:2475–2481, 1974.
54. Soli, N. E. and Froslie, A.: Chronic copper poisoning in sheep. I. The relationship of methaemoglobinemia to Heinz body formation and haemolysis during terminal crisis. Acta Pharmacol. Toxicol. *40*:169–177, 1977.
55. Adams, P. C., Strand, R. D., Bresnan, M. J., and Lucky, A. W.: Kinky hair syndrome: Serial study of radiological findings with emphasis on the similarity to the battered child syndrome. Radiology *112*:401–407, 1974.
56. Salhany, J. M., Swanson, J. C., Cordes, K. A., Gaines, S. B., and Gaines, K. C.: Evidence suggesting direct oxidation of human erythrocyte membrane sulfhydryls by copper. Biochem. Biophys. Res. Commun. *82*:1294–1299, 1978.
57. Nakashima, K., Fugii, S., and Kaneko, T.: Membrane protein cross-linking is an early step in the pathogenesis of copper-induced hemolytic anemia. Biomed. Res. *1*:548–551, 1980.
57a. Meyer, R. J., and Zalusky, R.: The mechanisms of hemolysis in Wilson's disease: study of a case and review of the literature. Mt. Sinai J. Med. *44*:532–538, 1977.
58. Sternlieb, I., and Goldfischer, S.: Heavy metals and lysosomes. *In* Lysosomes in Biology and Pathology. Vol. 5. Ed. by Dingle, J. T., and Dean, R. T. Elsevier, New York, 1976, pp. 185–200.
58a. Nagatsu, T., Kato, T., Nogatsu, I., Kondo, Y., Inga, K. S., Iizuka, R., and Narabayashi, H.: Catecholamine-related enzymes in the brain of patients with parkinsonism and Wilson's disease. Adv. Neurol. *24*:283–292, 1979.
58b. Nijeholt, J. L. A., and Korf, J.: Wilson's disease amd monoamines. Arch. Neurol. *35*:617, 1978.
59. Vogel, F. S., and Kemper, L.: *In vitro* acceleration of respiratory activity of neural tissues by copper. Lab. Invest. *10*:883–891, 1961.
59a. Cumpelik, O., and Paulin M.: Inhibition of mitochondrial monoamine oxidase by cadmium and copper. Naunyn-Schmiedeberg's Arch. Pharmacol. R23(Suppl. 307), 1979.
60. Prakash, N. J., Fontana, J., and Henkin, R. I.: Effect of transitional metal ions on ($Na^+ + K^+$) ATPase activity and the uptake of norepinephrine and choline by brain substrates. Life Sci. *12*:249–259, 1973.
61. Peters, R., and Walshe, J. M.: Studies on the toxicity of copper. I. The toxic action of copper *in vivo* and *in vitro*. Proc. Royal Soc. B *166*:273–284, 1966.
62. Peters, R., Shorthouse, M., and Walshe, J. M.: Studies on the toxicity of copper. II. The behaviour of microsomal membrane ATPase of the pigeon's brain tissue to copper and some other metallic substances. Proc. Royal Soc. B. *166*:285–294, 1966.
63. Baba, A., Kihara, T., Lee, E., and Iwata, H.: Activation of rat brain adenylate cyclase by copper plus dithiothreitol. Biochem. Pharmacol. *30*:171–174, 1981.
64. Komulainen, H., and Tuomisto, J.: Effect of copper on the uptake and release of monoamines in rat brain synatosomes. Acta Pharmacol. Toxicol. *48*:205–213, 1981.
65. Vogel, F. S., and Evans, J. W.: Morphologic alterations produced by copper in neural tissues with consideration of the role of the metal in the pathogenesis of Wilson's disease. J. Exp. Med. *113*:997–1004, 1961.
65a. Bal, H.: Effects of copper sulphate poisoning in white rats. Naturwiss. *51*:139, 1964.
66. Hernandez-Perez, O., Ballesteros, L. M., Mendez, D., and Rosado, A.: Accion disociante del cobre sobre les polisomas del hígado y del cerebro de la rata. Gaceta Med. Mexico *110*:205–211, 1975.
67. Johnson, R. A., and Sutherland, E. W.: Detergent-dispersed adenylate cyclase from rat brain. Effects of fluoride, cations and chelators. J. Biol. Chem. *248*:5114–5121, 1973.
68. Ting-Beall, H. P., Clark, D. A., Suelter, C. H., and Wells, W. W.: Studies on the interaction of chick brain microsomal ($Na^+ + K^+$)-ATPase with copper. Biochim. Biophys. Acta *291*:229–236, 1973.

69. Bowler, K., and Duncan, C. J.: The effect of copper on membrane enzymes. Biochim. Biophys. Acta *196*:116–119, 1970.
70. Donaldson, J., St.-Pierre, I., Minnich, J., and Barbeau, A.: Seizures in rats associated with divalent cation inhibition of Na^+-K^+-ATPase. Can. J. Biochem. *49*:1217–1224, 1971.
70a. Epstein. P. S., and McIlwain, H.: Actions of cupric salts on isolated cerebral tissues. Proc. Royal Soc. B. *166*:295–302, 1966.
71. Hexum, T. D.: Studies on the reaction catalyzed by transport (Na,K) adenosine triphosphatase I. Biochem. Pharmacol. *23*:3441–3447, 1974.
72. Marzullo, G., and Friedhoff, A. J.: An inhibitor of opiate receptor binding from human erythrocytes identified as a glutathione-copper complex. Life Sci. *21*:1559–1568, 1977.
73. Nathanson, J. A., and Bloom, F. E.: Heavy metals and adenosine cyclic 3′5′-monophosphate metabolism: Possible relevance to heavy metal toxicity. Mol. Pharmacol. *12*:390–398, 1976.
74. Heikkila, R. E., and Cabbat, F. S.: The stimulation of 6–hydroxydopamine autoxidation by divalent copper: potential importance in the neurotoxic process. Life Sci. *23*:33–38, 1978.
75. Victor, M.: Neurologic changes in liver disease. *In* Brain Dysfunction in Metabolic Disorders, Vol. 53. Ed. by Plum, F. Raven Press, New York, 1974, pp. 1–12.
75a. Anonymous: The astrocyte in liver disease. Lancet *II*:1189–1190, 1971.
76. Voinar, A. I., and Galakhova, V. N.: Effect of copper on the glycogen and lipid contents of the liver. Ukr. Biokhim. Zh. *34*:505–506, 1962.
76a. Grabske, R. J.: The effect of Cu^{2+} on oxidative phosphorylation and the structural stability of isolated mitochondria. J. Cell Biol. *35*:48–49A, 1967.
77. Barka, T., Scheuer, P. J., Schaffner, F., and Popper, H.: Structural changes of liver cells in copper intoxication. Arch. Pathol. *78*:331–349, 1964.
78. Hernandez, O., Ballesteros, L. M., Mendez, J. D., and Rosado, A.: Copper as a dissociating agent of liver and endometrial polysomes. Fertil. Steril. *25*:108–112, 1974.
79. Moffit, A. E., Jr., and Murphy, S. D.: Effect of excess and deficient copper intake on rat liver microsomal enzyme activity. Biochem. Pharmacol. *22*:1463–1476, 1973.
80. Parkki, M. G.: Effect of methyl mercury p-chloromercurobenzoate and dimethyl cadmium on rat hepatic epoxide hydrase *in vitro*. Toxicol. Lett. *3*:166a, 1980.
81. Mize, C. E., and Langdon, R. G.: Hepatic glutathione reductase. I. Purification and general kinetic properties. J. Biol. Chem. *237*:1589–1595, 1962.

CHAPTER 5

PATHOLOGY OF THE LIVER

The histologic abnormalities seen in a single biopsy specimen taken from any one patient with Wilson's disease are rarely, if ever, pathognomonic of this disorder. What is unique, however, is the sequential development that can be derived from observations of several biopsy samples taken from individual patients serially over years; or of single samples from each of many patients at different phases of the evolution of the hepatic lesion. Then the progression of the pathologic picture, from one in which hepatocytic glycogen nuclei and narrow bands of portal fibrosis are the only deviations from normality to end-stage mixed micronodular and macronodular cirrhosis, can be appreciated. In the course of carrying out such a study quantitative copper analyses were made on most biopsy specimens, revealing an excess of the metal (ranging from five to fifty times the normal maximum of 50 mcg/g dry liver) in about 97 per cent of untreated patients. (We have discussed, in Chapter 4, why younger patients, with minimal or moderate pathologic changes, have considerably higher hepatic copper concentrations than the older patients with established cirrhosis and advanced Wilson's disease—see Fig. 4–1.)

GROSS PATHOLOGIC FINDINGS

During infancy the color and appearance of the liver of a patient with Wilson's disease are normal. When fatty infiltration, the first frank histopathologic event, is present, the liver is usually pale, enlarged and smooth. As chronic hepatitis develops, the liver may shrink and show accentuated lobular markings. It becomes brownish or green as it progresses to the final stage of nodular cirrhosis[1–13] (Fig. 5–1). Then splenomegaly[14, 15]; esophageal varices; collateral venous channels[16, 17]; ascites, occasionally with spontaneous bacterial peritonitis[18]; thrombosis of the portal vein[19]; aneurysms of the splenic artery[20]; or combinations of these and other features of portal hypertension are seen. Except, perhaps, for an increased incidence of cholelithiasis,[21, 22] the biliary system is usually normal.

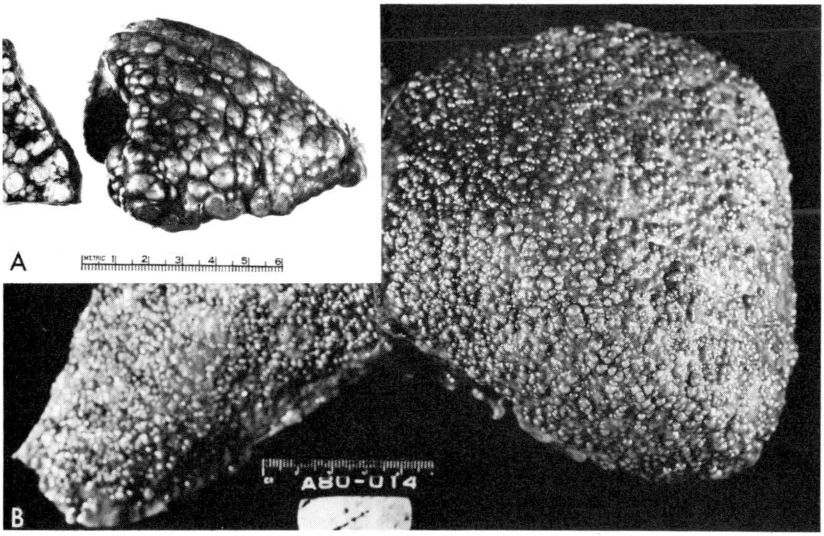

Figure 5–1. Mixed micronodular and macronodular cirrhosis (**A**, a 16-year-old boy, F4) or micronodular cirrhosis (**B**, a 15-year-old boy, P1) are seen in these autopsy specimens of liver from patients with advanced Wilson's disease.

LIGHT MICROSCOPIC FINDINGS

In our laboratory we have assessed, microscopically, the hepatic appearance of more than 200 patients with Wilson's disease: *None was normal*. For many years we believed that a biopsy specimen from a 3½-year-old boy, G3, was an exception, because his hepatocytes appeared normal to light microscopy, except for the presence of chiefly periportal, glycogen-filled, ballooned nuclei, which, though the earliest and most frequently encountered hepatocellular abnormality, are only arguably pathologic. But re-examination of the specimen, which contained 1092 mcg/g dry liver, revealed unmistakable portal fibrosis (Fig. 5–2).

Fatty changes—unequivocally pathologic—are first manifest as fine lipid droplets, shown to be composed of triglycerides when frozen sections are stained with oil red O.[4–6, 23, 24] They are the most commonly found abnormalities in young asymptomatic patients, but they are not present in the liver biopsy specimens obtained from age-matched heterozygous carriers, in whom the light microscopic findings are usually entirely normal. The lipid droplets increase in numbers and size with time, metamorphosing into hepatic steatosis resembling that caused by ethanol, occasionally with lipid granulomas in portal tracts or lobules (Fig. 5–3).

The lesion then expands with hyperplasia of Kupffer cells, small infiltrates of mononuclear cells, further deposition of pericellular and periportal collagen with formation of intralobular septa extending from the portal tracts (Figs. 5–4 and 5–5) and development of fibrosis around the central vein. These early phases may progress to cirrhosis silently; to acute, sometimes clinically fulminant, hepatitis; or through a stage of chronic active hepatitis.

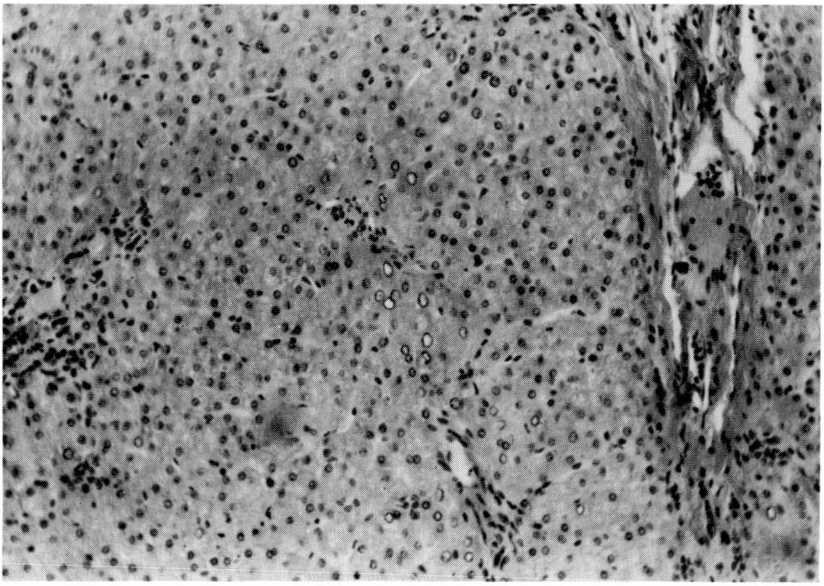

Figure 5–2. Normal lobular architecture and hepatocytes, except for ballooned glycogen nuclei, in the periportal zone. There are excess collagen deposits in the periportal and pericentral areas. Biopsy specimen containing 1092 mcg copper/g dry liver. 3½-year-old asymptomatic boy, G3. Hematoxylin-eosin. × 120.

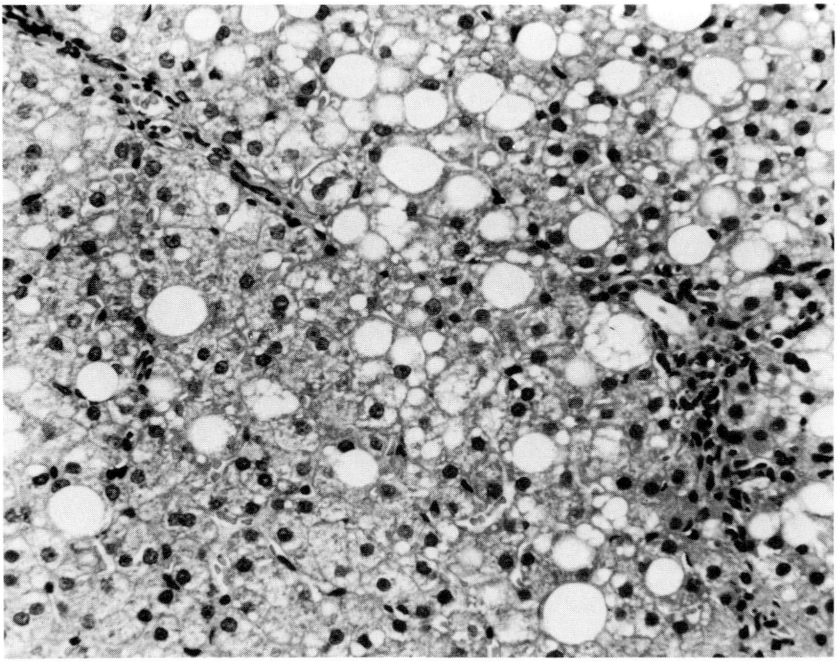

Figure 5–3. Some of the earliest pathologic findings visible by light microscopy include irregular-appearing hepatocytes with lipid droplets of varying sizes, prominent Kupffer cells, moderate cellular infiltrates and a slender fibrous band. Needle biopsy specimen. 1158 mcg copper/g dry liver. 6-year-old asymptomatic boy, P8. Hematoxylin-eosin. × 250.

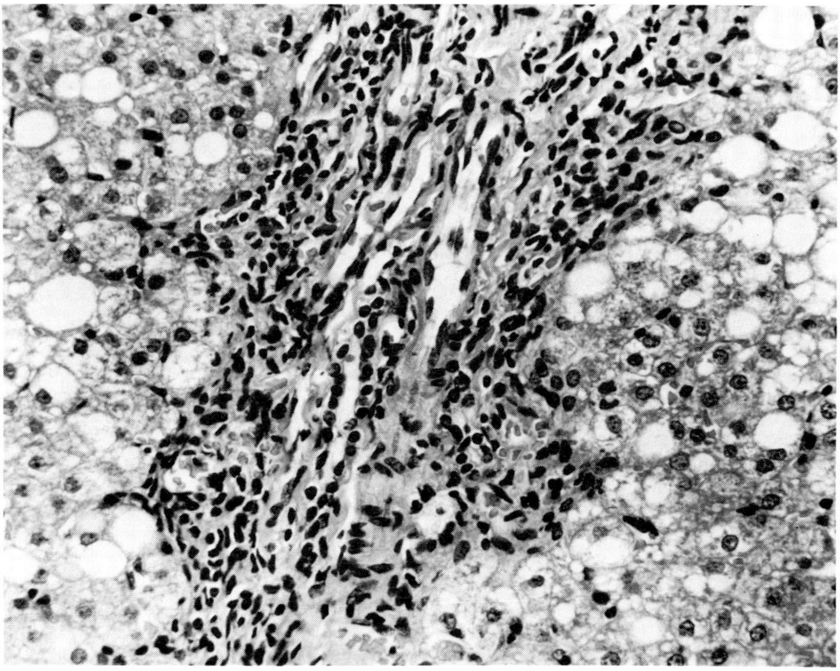

Figure 5–4. More pronounced cellular infiltrate spilling through the marginal plate and isolating individual hepatocytes in another portion of the same biopsy specimen shown in Figure 5–3. Deposition of collagen is heavier. Hematoxylin-eosin. × 250.

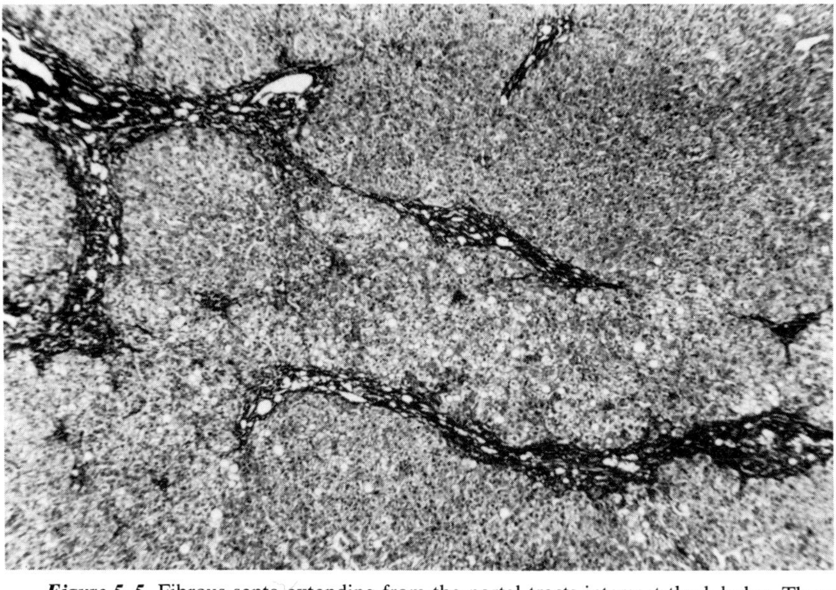

Figure 5–5. Fibrous septa extending from the portal tracts intersect the lobules. There is only mild steatosis, but no collapse, inflammation or cirrhosis. Surgical biopsy. 1710 mcg copper/g dry liver. 19-year-old asymptomatic man, S8. Trichrome. × 160.

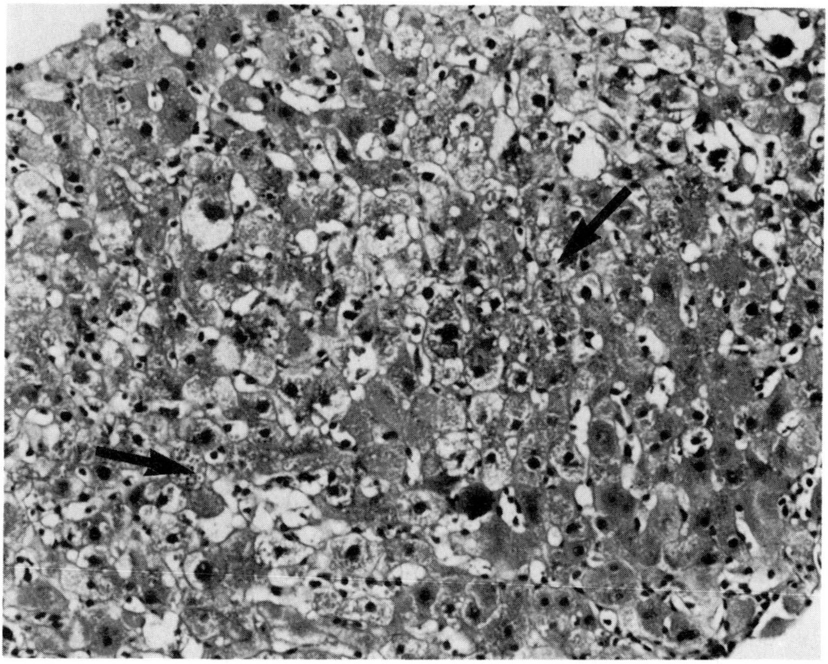

Figure 5–6. Irregularly shaped hepatocytes, many of them ballooned, containing clumped, eosinophilic cytoplasm or microvesicular lipid vacuoles and irregularly appearing nuclei suggestive of a cytotoxic process. Intracellular cholestasis *(arrows)*; prominent Kupffer cells; few inflammatory cells. Needle biopsy specimen. 941 mcg copper/g dry liver. 19-year-old woman, F5, suffering from an acute episode of hemolytic jaundice. Hematoxylin-eosin. × 375.

Liver biopsy, though rarely performed during the acute hepatitis of Wilson's disease (since the illness is almost always thought to be infectious hepatitis), yields tissue characterized by cytoplasmic swelling; eosinophilic clumping and necrosis of hepatocytes, with sparse lymphocytic infiltrations, acidophilic or Councilman bodies in various portions of the lobules; and cholestasis (Fig. 5–6).

If florid chronic active hepatitis develops, any combination of the following abnormalities may be seen: ballooning of hepatocytes, anisocytosis, eosinophilic clumping of hepatocytic cytoplasm, focal necrosis associated mainly with histiocytic cells, anisokaryosis, binucleated or trinucleated hepatocytes, glycogen accumulations or cytoplasmic invaginations into nuclei, prominent infiltrates containing round cells and segmented leukocytes, erosion of marginal plates, proliferated bile ductules surrounded by inflammatory cells and fibrous tissue, and cirrhosis (Figs. 5–7 and 5–8). The last, despite the relative brevity of the clinical disease, is more often seen than not.

The phase of chronic hepatitis may subside spontaneously or escalate suddenly into pathologically subacute disease that clinically may mimic fulminant hepatitis (see Chapter 7). This stage of the disease is characterized by microvesicular fat, coagulative cell necrosis,[11] occasional giant and multinucleated cells, large pigment-laden Kupffer cells, stroma-collapse,

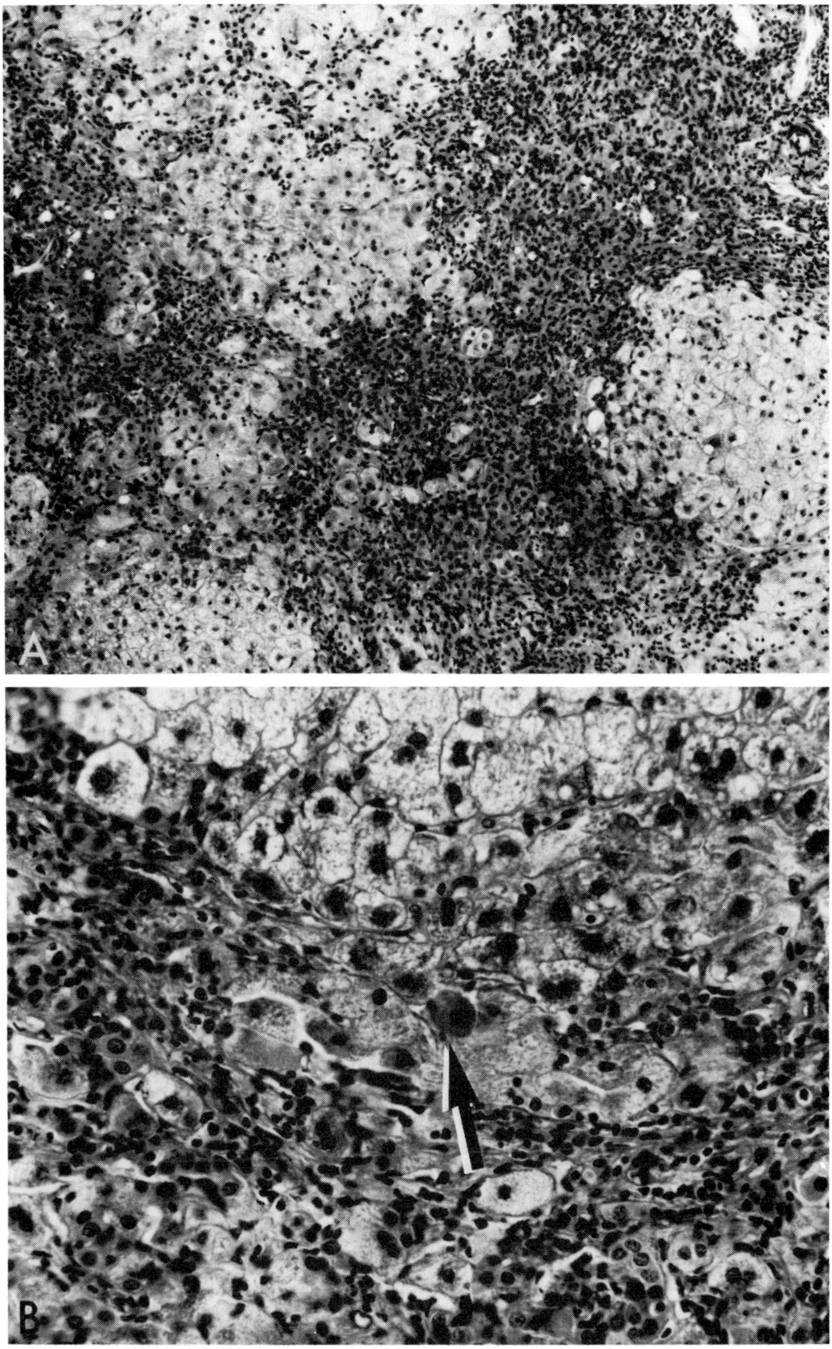

Figure 5–7. Appearance of "chronic active hepatitis" with distortion of lobular architecture, heavy inflammatory infiltrates and isolation of hepatocytes by infiltrates of round cells and histiocytes. The hepatocytes vary in size and show cytoplasmic degeneration and ballooning. There are scattered acidophilic bodies *(arrow)*. Surgical liver biopsy specimen. 971 mcg copper/g dry liver. 12-year-old boy, B1, who was previously healthy, presented with acute hemolytic jaundice and evidence of hepatic dysfunction and splenomegaly. Hematoxylin-eosin. **A,** × 100; **B,** × 250.

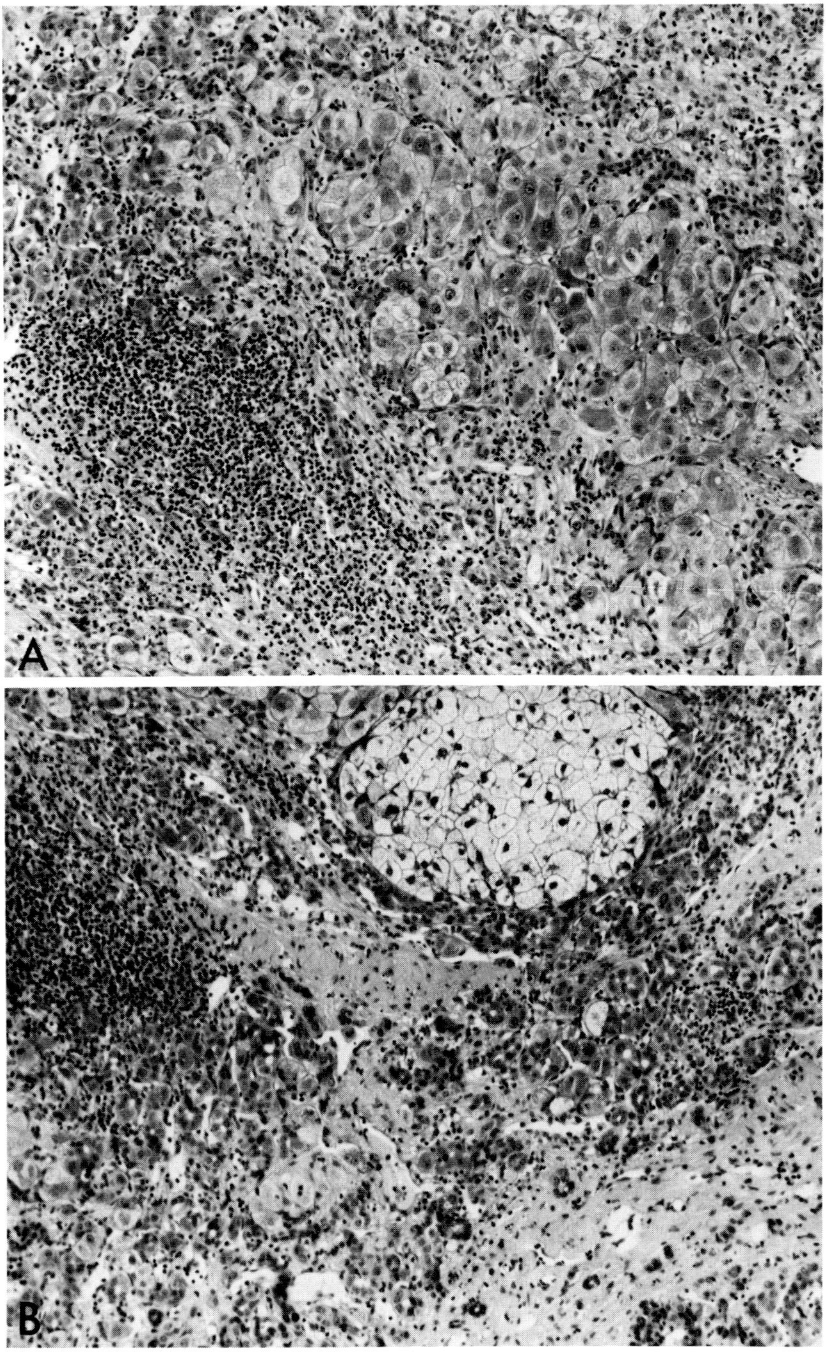

Figure 5–8. Appearance of "chronic active hepatitis" with disorganization of the normal lobular architecture and infiltration of round cells through the marginal plates in **A**. In **B** there are regenerating nodules and broad fibrous bands, together indicative of cirrhosis. Surgical liver biopsy specimen. 1422 mcg copper/g dry liver. 10-year-old boy, G4, with recent onset of ascites and a serum bilirubin of 4.3 mg/dl. Hematoxylin-eosin. × 110.

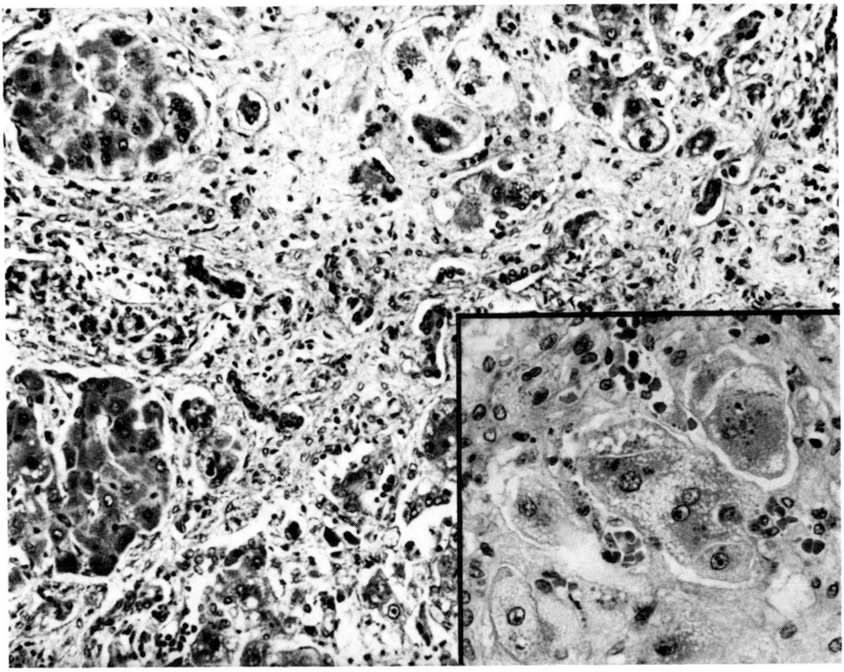

Figure 5–9. Submassive collapse of parenchyma with a few residual islets of hepatocytes and scattered, profoundly altered hepatocytes showing enlargement and eosinophilic clumping. Autopsy specimen of liver. 1153 mcg copper/g dry liver. A 20-year-old college student, A1, died six weeks after an insidious onset of jaundice with hemolysis, rapidly progressing to hepatic and renal failure, and mimicking fulminant hepatitis. Kayser-Fleischer rings were discovered four days before a sudden respiratory arrest. Trichrome. × 150. *Inset*: Hematoxylin-eosin. × 250.

and Mallory's cytoplasmic hyalin, predominantly in peripheral, residual hepatocytes[23] (Fig. 5–9). These findings differ from the large eosinophilic hepatocytes, segmented leukocytes and large Kupffer cells devoid of ceroid seen at the corresponding stage of viral hepatitis.

Ultimately, whatever the course, there is cirrhosis, with slender or broad fibrous bands composed mostly of Types I and III collagen[11a] separating regenerating nodules. In some patients the abnormal collagen deposits in the subintimal layers of central and sublobular veins resemble veno-occlusive disease with endophlebitis and infiltrations (predominantly by lymphocytes) of the vessel wall.[11]

The ratios of the two types of collagen seen in three patients whose livers were so analyzed were probably affected by the penicillamine they had received. One of these patients, M2, treated for 8 years, showed a markedly reduced content of Type III collagen, a finding to be expected from the effect of penicillamine in inhibiting cross-linking of Type I collagen.[11b]

In the cirrhotic liver the hepatocytes may be arranged in a pseudoductular array. They may display only minimal cytologic alterations or nuclear "unrest." The nodules may also contain mononuclear infiltrates

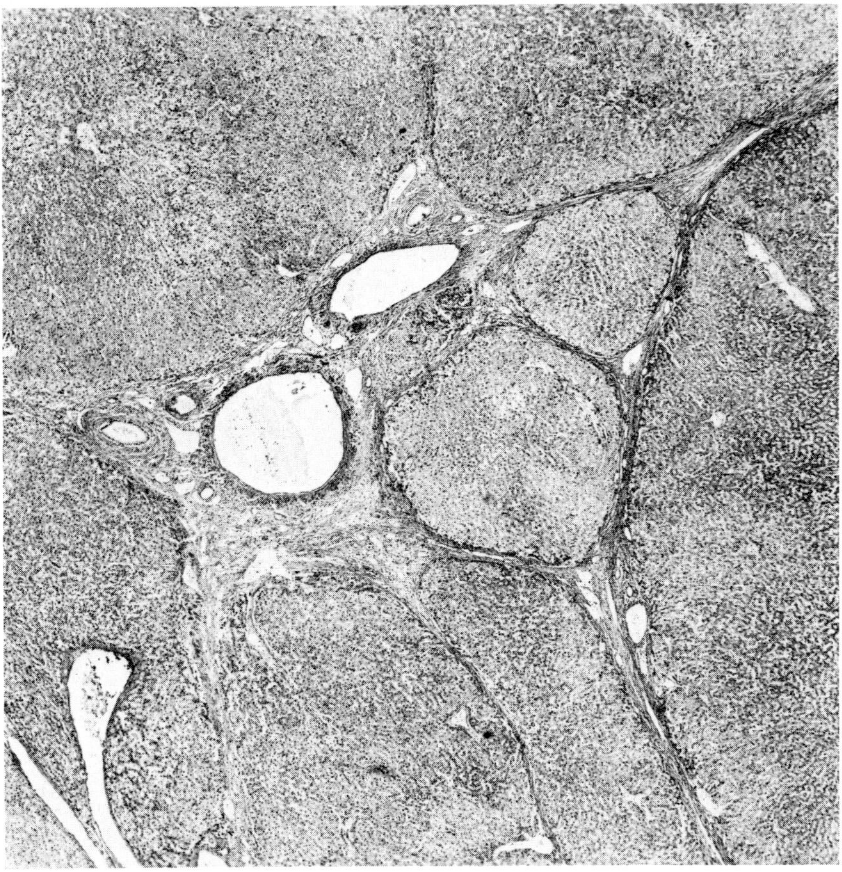

Figure 5–10. Irregularly sized nodules of hepatic parenchyma are separated by fine bands of fibrous tissue. Autopsy specimen of liver. 515 mcg copper/g dry liver. This 24-year-old woman, M2, first presented with anasarca, mild jaundice and dysarthria at age 16 years. With D-penicillamine treatment there was significant improvement in liver function and speech. She died of her third exsanguinating hemorrhage from ruptured esophageal varices. Hematoxylin-eosin. × 28.

that vary in size according to the stage of activity of the inflammatory process, some eosinophils and an abundance of proliferated bile ductules in the fibrous septa (Figs. 5–10 and 5–11), as well as an increased number of capillaries.[11] In some nodules there may be excess fat and hepatocytic glycogen nuclei, invaginations of cytoplasm into nuclei, an increase in binucleated and trinucleated cells or leukocytic infiltrates. Granules, fine or coarse, are prominent in the hepatocytes, particularly in the periportal areas.[11, 23] They may contain lipofuscin pigment, "copper-associated protein," acid phosphatase, or, occasionally, iron.[23a] If the pathologic process cannot be arrested, extensive collapse, hepatocellular degeneration (with retained bile pigment) and necrosis lead to hepatic insufficiency and death from exsanguination, sepsis, endotoxemia, hepatorenal syndrome or encephalopathy.

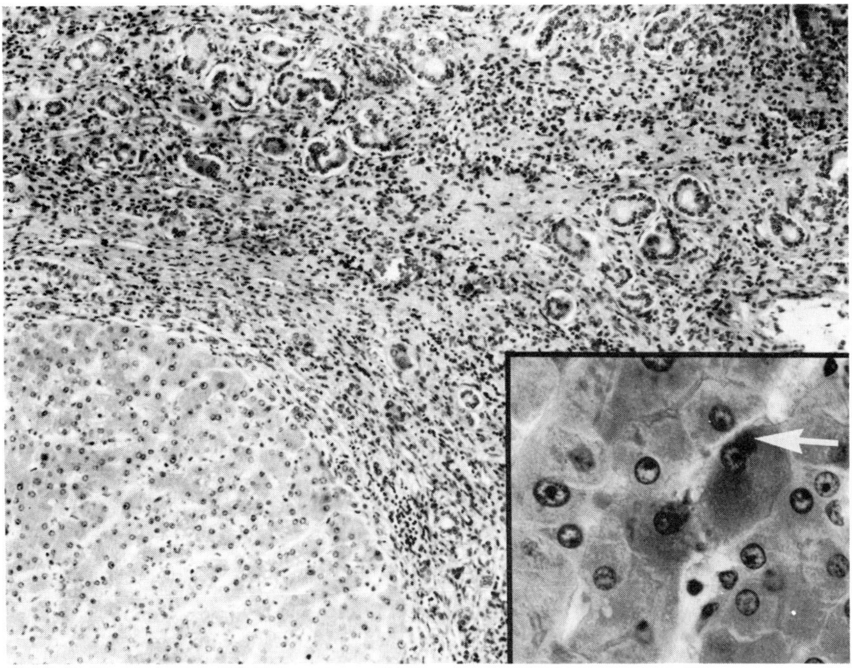

Figure 5–11. Moderate round and polymorphonuclear cell infiltrates and broad bands of fibrous tissue, with numerous proliferating bile ductules, outline the regenerating nodules in this cirrhotic liver with partial collapse of parenchyma. Autopsy specimen. 18 mcg copper/g dry liver. A 22-year-old woman, R4, who first presented, at 18, with primary amenorrhea and clinical and laboratory evidence of hepatic dysfunction. Suspected of suffering from chronic hepatitis, the diagnosis of Wilson's disease was made only after the appearance of ascites, neurologic and psychiatric symptoms two years later. At her death, of hepatic insufficiency, the liver was shrunken and cirrhotic. Hematoxylin-eosin. × 100. *Inset:* Mallory body *(arrow)*. × 400.

HISTOCHEMISTRY AND CYTOCHEMISTRY

Copper may be stained in histologic sections with rhodanine,[25–27] rubeanic acid[28–30] or Timm's silver sulfide.[30–32] These stains, like electron probe microanalysis,[33] although only qualitative estimates of the liver's copper content, are of great value in determining the lobular, nodular and intracellular distribution of copper. Sipponen has found that orcein stains the poorly characterized copper-associated protein, rich in sulfhydryl groups and located within hepatocellular granules,[34] which also stain with Victoria blue. In ultraviolet light these granules exhibit golden-brown fluorescence[6] (as does the lysosomal copper-protein isolated from the livers of Bedlington terriers with inherited hepatic copper toxicosis[34]) and stain with oil red O, Nile blue,[6] the periodic acid–Schiff procedure after diastase treatment, Schmorl's ferro-ferricyanide reaction for reducing substances and Fontana's stain—all indicative of the presence of lipofuscin.[11, 25] These granules are lysosomes, since they also contain acid phosphatase demonstrable by staining[28, 31] and by electron probe microanalysis.[33]

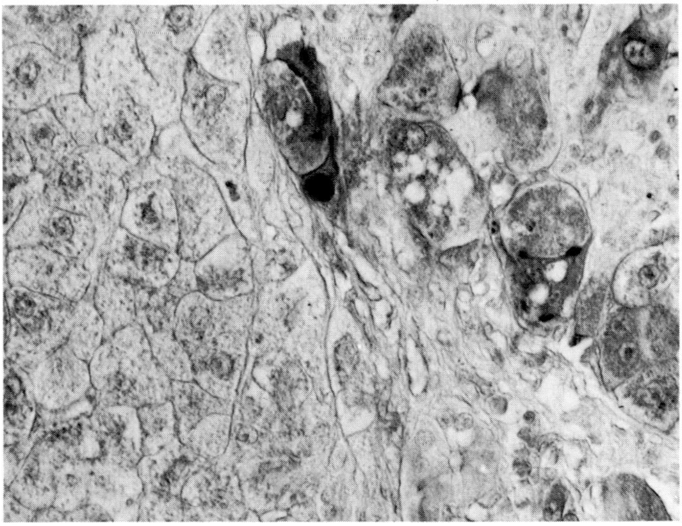

Figure 5–12. Copper is diffuse, finely granular and uniformly stained over certain hepatocytes that show some fatty changes *(F)*. Needle biopsy specimen. 507 mcg copper/g dry tissue. 11-year-old asymptomatic girl, S18. Paraffin section, Timm's silver sulfide stain. × 600. (Courtesy Dr. Sidney Goldfischer.)

The intracellular distribution of copper differs markedly in early and late Wilson's disease. During the early stages of Wilson's disease, when the hepatic concentrations of copper are at their highest, copper, paradoxically, is detectable histochemically and cytochemically only by very sensitive stains, such as Timm's silver sulfide. The copper, in this stage of the disease, is diffusely distributed in the cytoplasm of hepatocytes[31] (Fig. 5–12), so that its concentration at any point in the cell is much lower than late in the disease, when the metal is almost all within lysosomes and is detectable by such relatively insensitive stains as rubeanic acid or rhodanine. Therefore, absence of copper staining does not exclude the diagnosis at the time when it is the most difficult to make and of greatest value to the patient—*early* in Wilson's disease.[25, 31–33, 35]

In the advanced stages hepatocytes with copper-containing, orcein-positive granules are present almost throughout certain nodules yet are absent from others (Fig. 5–13). This distribution of copper is characteristic of Wilson's disease, and differs from the distribution of copper-laden hepatocytes predominantly at the periphery of most lobules or nodules in the livers of many patients with advanced primary biliary cirrhosis or cholestasis.[25, 36–38]

Mallory's cytoplasmic hyaline, found in the livers of some patients dying after a subacutely progressive course, has been shown immunocytochemically to be identical to that present in other forms of severe liver disease.[39] Occasionally, excessive iron deposits are seen in hepatocytes stained with Perl's stain.[23a] Neither intracellular alpha-1-antitrypsin, on PAS-stained sections, or hepatitis B surface antigen, following aldehyde fuchsin staining, has been seen.[11]

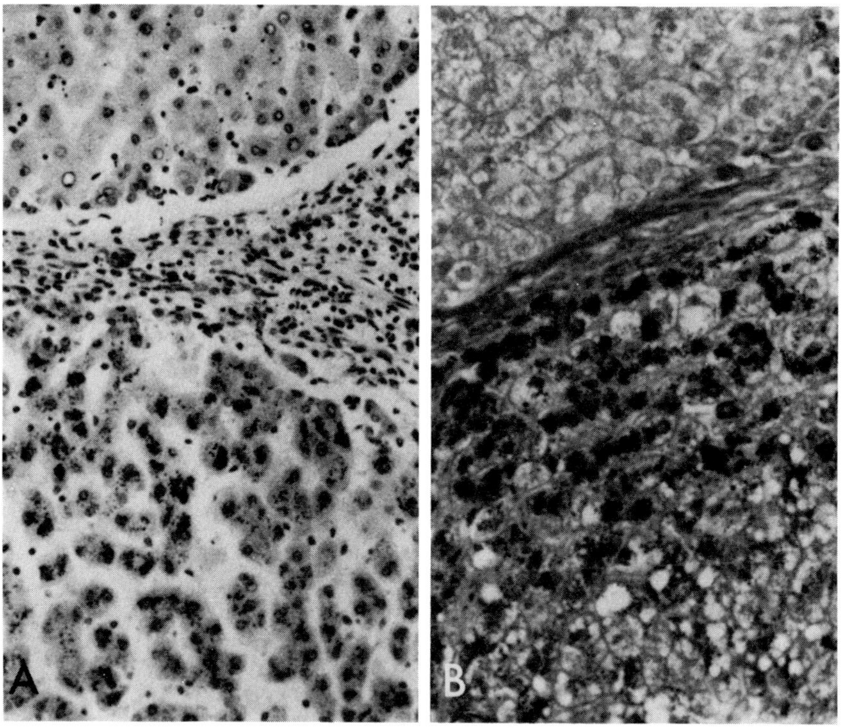

Figure 5–13. Almost all hepatocytes in one nodule stain for copper contained in granules (**A**) and for copper-associated protein (**B**), whereas adjacent nodules are unstained. Serial sections of surgical biopsy specimen. 971 mcg copper/g dry liver. Patient B1 (see Figure 5–7). **A**, Rhodanine; **B**, orcein. × 60. (From Goldfischer, S., Popper, H., and Sternlieb, I.: Amer. J. Pathol. *99*:715–730, 1980, with permission.)

ELECTRON MICROSCOPY

Wilson's disease is one of the few liver diseases in which there are pathognomonic ultrastructural changes. In the earliest stages of fatty infiltration, hepatocellular mitochondria are often markedly pleomorphic and abnormally large, and they exhibit increased matrix density. The normally apposed inner and outer mitochondrial membranes separate and create intermembranous spaces; intercristal spaces widen; and large granules and crystalline, vacuolated or dense inclusions appear in the matrix[40–43] (Figs. 5–14 to 5–16). These abnormal mitochondria—*seen in no other condition*—disappear spontaneously with progression of the pathologic process toward cirrhosis.[40] In treated patients their rate of disappearance seems to be accelerated, as shown by a morphometric study.[44]

In some specimens the peroxisomes (organelles also involved in cellular lipid metabolism) are grossly abnormal: They become enlarged, rounded or misshapen, with a granular or flocculent matrix of varying electron density replacing the normal homogeneous one[45] (Figs. 5–17 and 5–18). When these peroxisomal changes are observed in fatty hepatocytes, very few mitochondrial abnormalities are seen.

Text continued on page 55

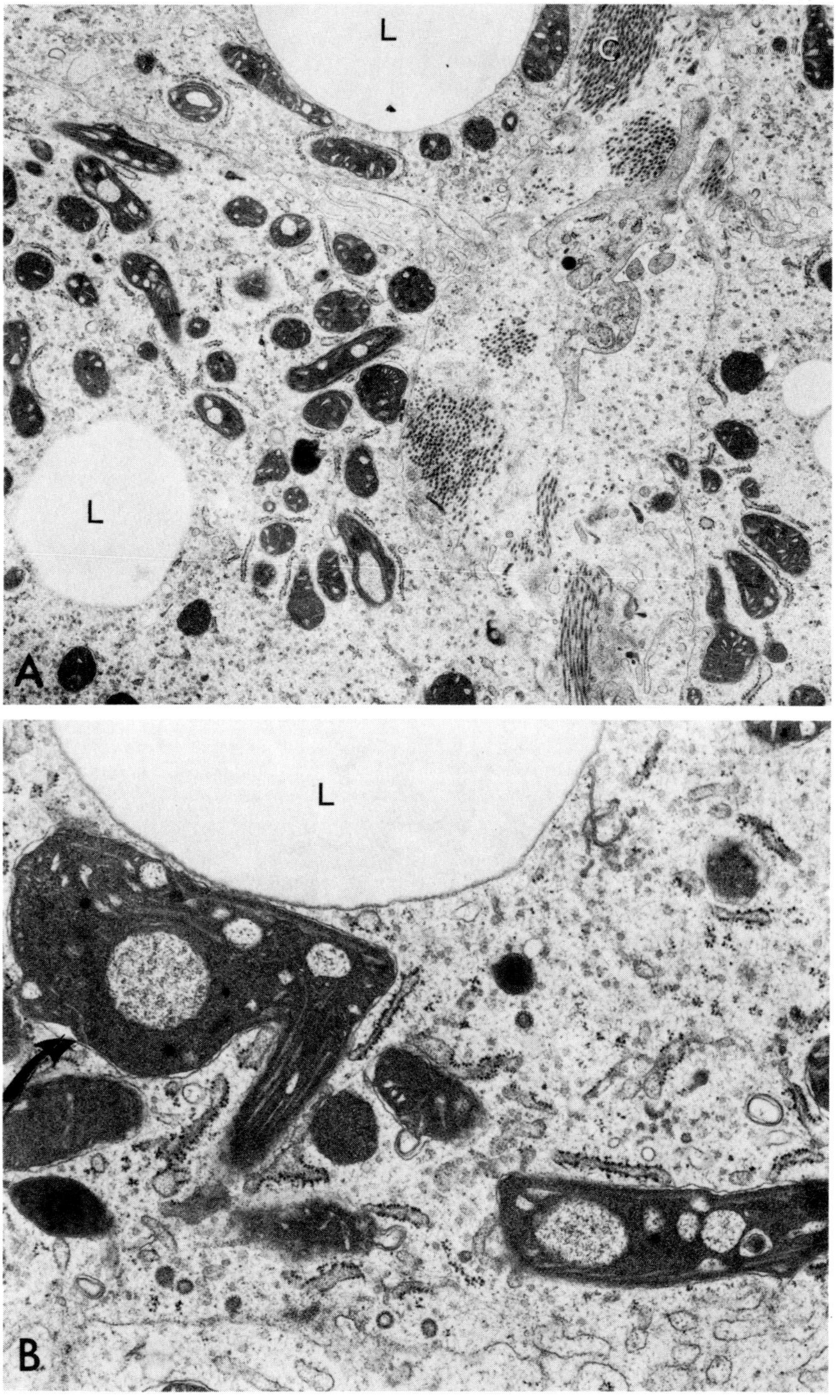

Figure 5–14. **A**, Portions of four hepatocytes containing lipid droplets *(L)* and abnormal mitochondria (see text), with bundles of collagen *(C)* in intercellular spaces. **B**, At a higher magnification there are abnormally dense matrices, separations of outer from inner membranes *(arrows)*, dilated cristae and vacuoles in mitochondria. Electron micrograph; needle biopsy specimen. 991 mcg copper/g dry liver. 5-year-old asymptomatic girl, G5. **A**, × 8100; **B,** × 15,000.

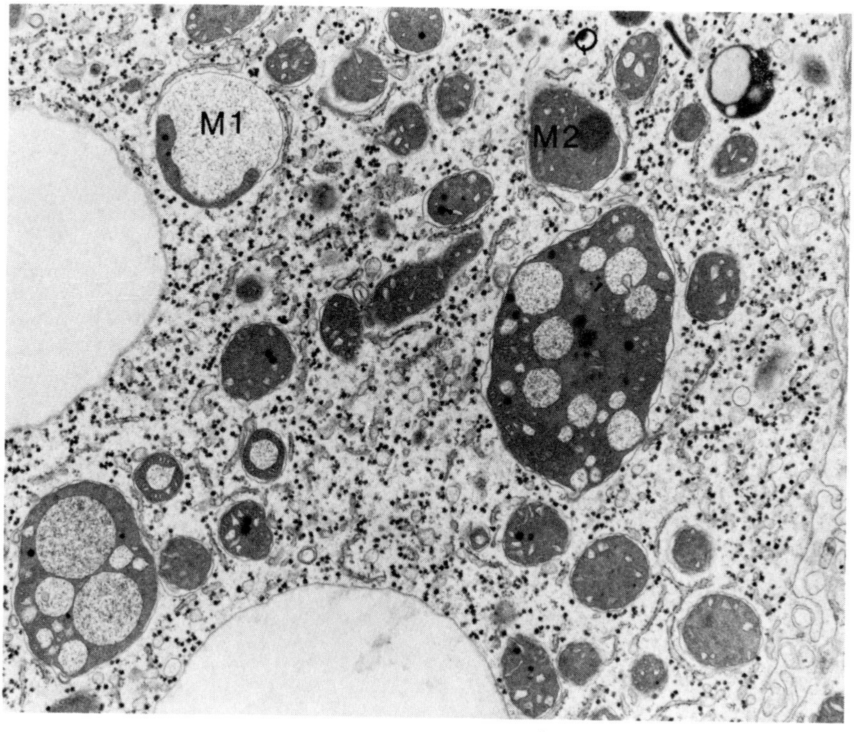

Figure 5–15. Grossly abnormal hepatocytic mitochondria. The matrix of mitochondrion M1 is almost entirely replaced by granular material. M2 contains a prominent dense inclusion. The endoplasmic reticulum and glycogen granules are unremarkable. Electron micrograph; needle biopsy specimen. 1029 mcg copper/g dry liver. 10-year-old asymptomatic girl, O2. × 9000.

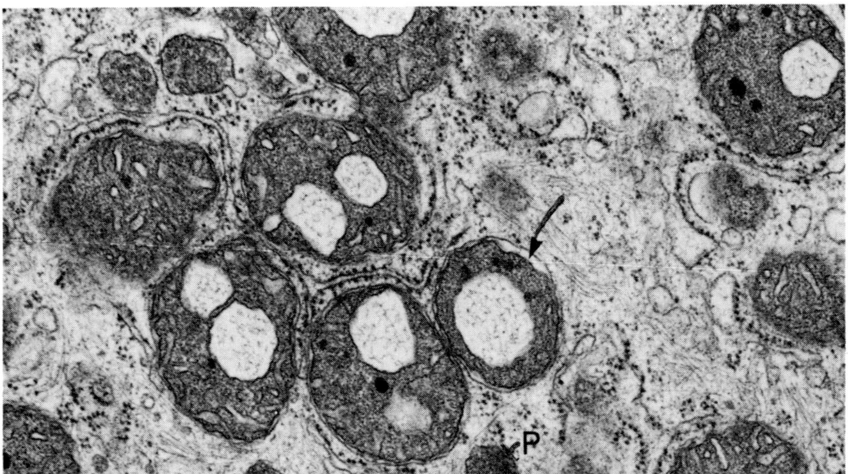

Figure 5–16. Mitochondria with large vacuoles and separation of membranes *(arrow)* in a portion of an hepatocyte. The peroxisomes *(P)* are smaller than normal, and there is an excess of filaments in the cytoplasm. Electron micrograph; needle biopsy specimen. 657 mcg copper/g dry liver. 10-year-old asymptomatic boy, S10. × 36,000.

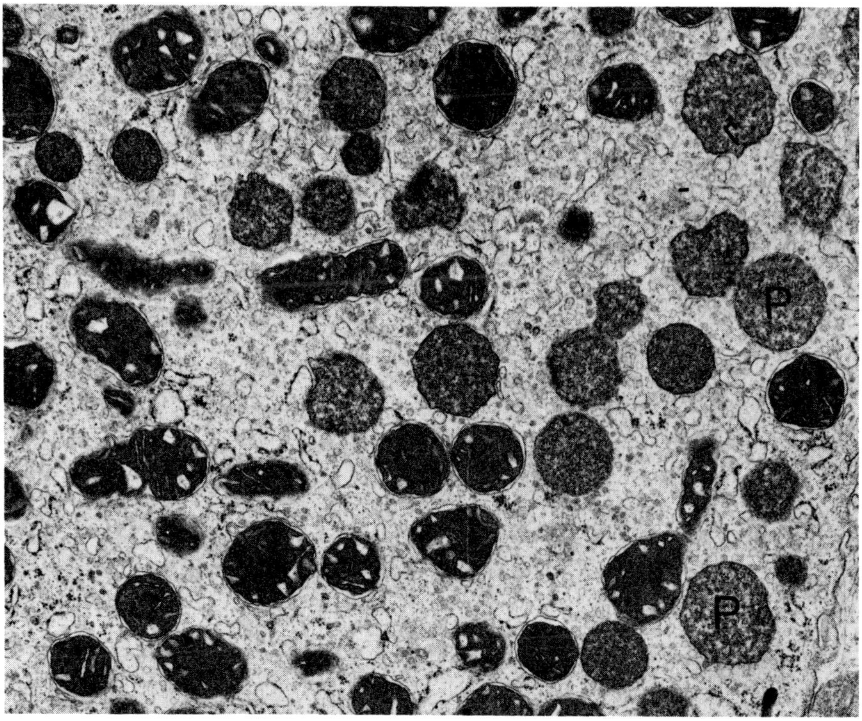

Figure 5–17. Abundant, irregularly shaped peroxisomes *(P)* with granular matrices next to abnormal mitochondria in another hepatocyte of the biopsy sample of Figure 5–15. Electron micrograph. × 14,800.

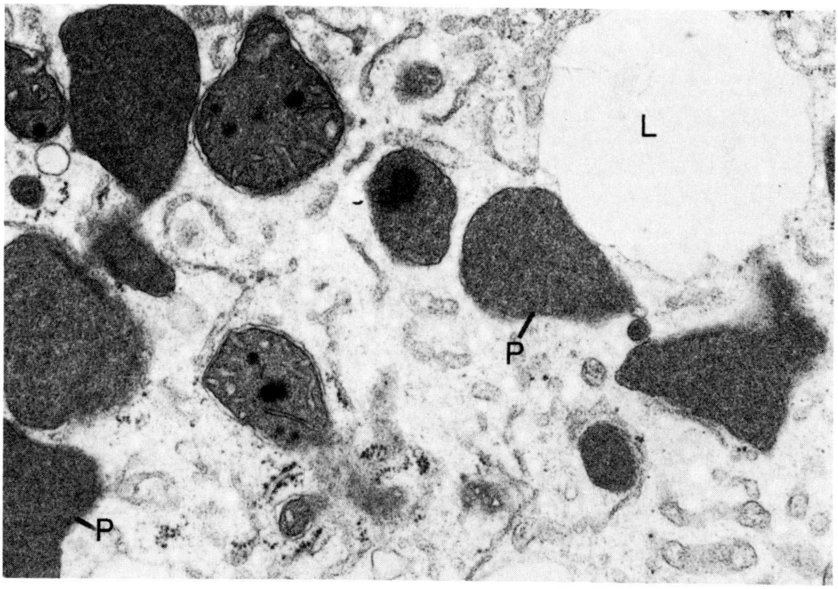

Figure 5–18. Peroxisomes *(P)* displaying more pronounced abnormalities than those illustrated in Figure 5–17. They are enlarged, irregularly shaped and dense, and contain occasional electron dense inclusions. *L,* lipid droplet. Electron micrograph; needle biopsy specimen. 912 mcg copper/g dry liver. 8-year-old asymptomatic boy, B2. × 16,900.

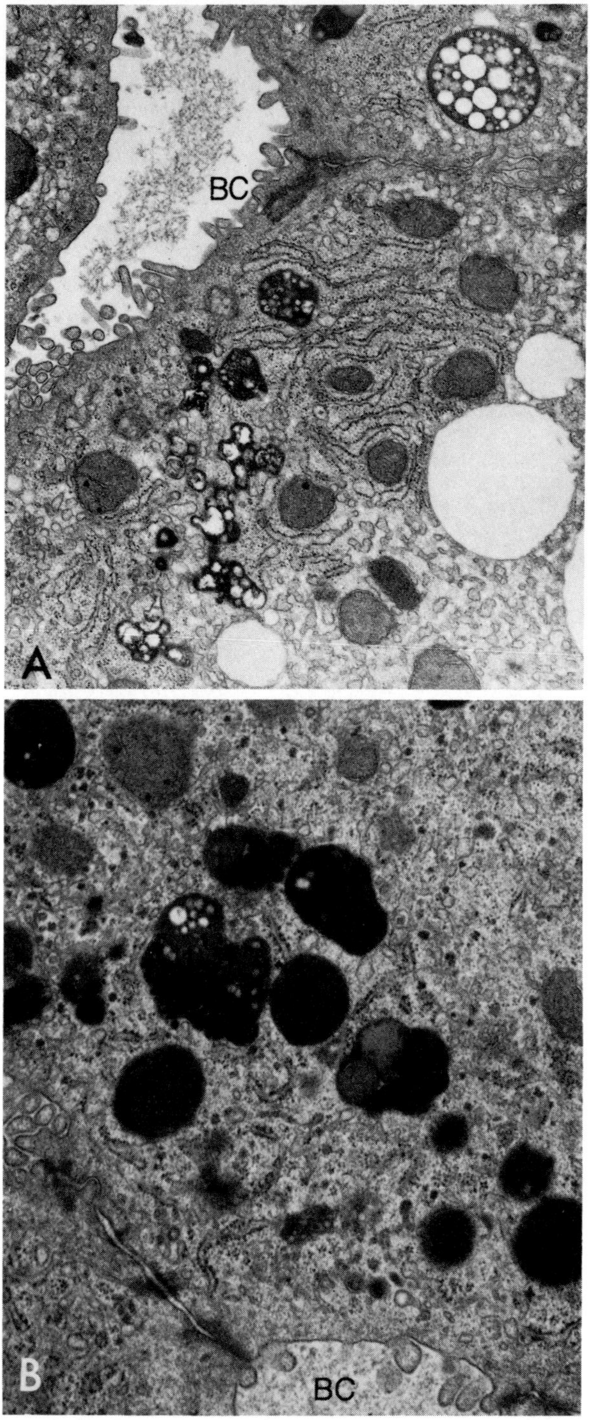

Figure 5–19. Heterogeneous, polymorphic bodies of variable electron density near the biliary poles of hepatocytes. These granules contain lipofuscin, copper and copper-associated protein. Electron micrograph; needle biopsy specimens. **A**, 14-year-old boy, E3, with psychiatric and neurologic manifestations and Kayser-Fleischer rings; **B**, 35-year-old man, S11, with neurologic Wilson's disease and Kayser-Fleischer rings. *BC*, biliary canaliculus. **A**, × 10,600; **B**, × 18,500.

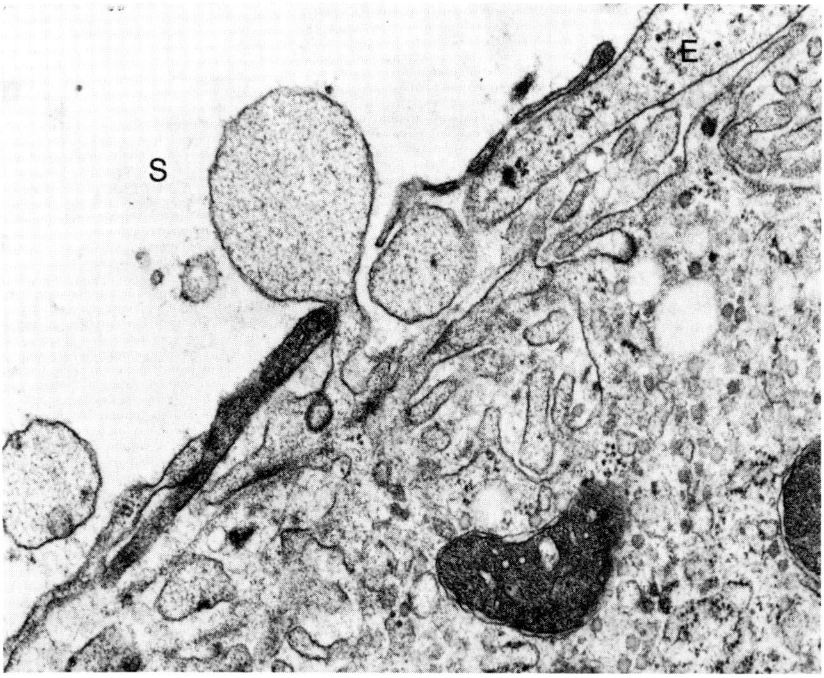

Figure 5–20. Cytoplasmic blebs project from the sinusoidal portion of an hepatocyte through the fenestrae of the sinusoidal endothelium. The mitochondria are only slightly abnormal. Electron micrograph; needle biopsy specimen. 1189 mcg copper/g dry liver. 13-year-old asymptomatic girl, T2. *E*, endothelial cell; *S*, sinusoid. × 22,200.

By the time cirrhosis has developed, the electron microscopic appearance of individual hepatocytes is almost normal except for abundant amorphous or globular lipofuscin granules[31, 32, 46–50] (Fig. 5–19), lipolysosomes,[51] and the occasional coexistence of both "light" and "dark" hepatocytes.

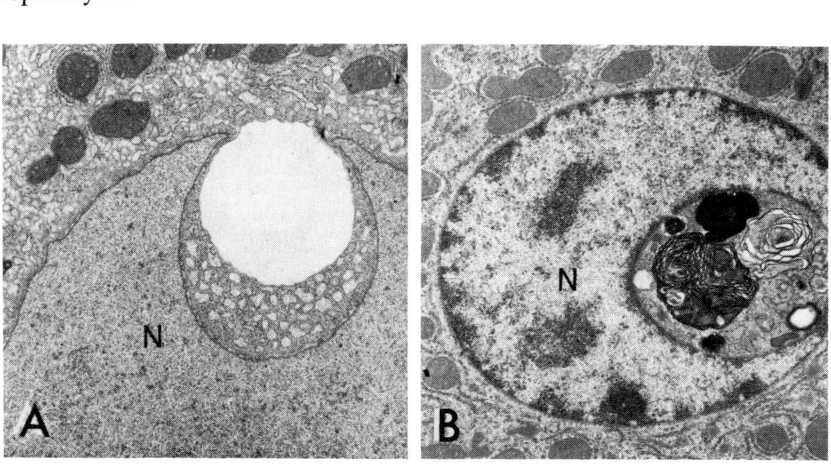

Figure 5–21. Invaginated cytoplasm in the nuclei *(N)* of hepatocytes. Electron micrographs; needle biopsy specimen. **A**, An 11-year-old girl, D5, and **B**, a 15-year-old adolescent boy, P9, both with asymptomatic Wilson's disease. × 6500.

In addition, in Wilson's disease, there are many nonspecific abnormalities of the fine structure of the liver recognizable under the electron microscope. These include formations of sinusoidal blebs (Fig. 5–20), which suggest injury to the plasma membrane; invaginations of the cytoplasm into nuclei of hepatocytes (Fig. 5–21); deposition of collagen fibrils or basement membrane material in Disse's space; abnormal separation of hepatocytes (Fig. 5–22); and pseudoglandular formations—all of which may be seen in other cirrhotic specimens. One may also find cytoplasmic crystals, proliferation of the endoplasmic reticulum (sometimes with fingerprint- or whorl-like structures) and fibrillar accumulations characteristic of Mallory bodies (Fig. 5–23.)[40, 52–54]

The livers of five siblings, three (S12, S13, and S14) in one family and two (S10 and S15) in another, were biopsied at approximately the same stage of Wilsonian hepatic steatosis. Although the pattern of the pathognomonic mitochondrial abnormalities was similar in each set of sibs, there were distinguishable differences between the two families—perhaps coincidental, perhaps reflecting unknown genetic factors affecting the severity of mitochondrial reactions to excess cytoplasmic copper.[55]

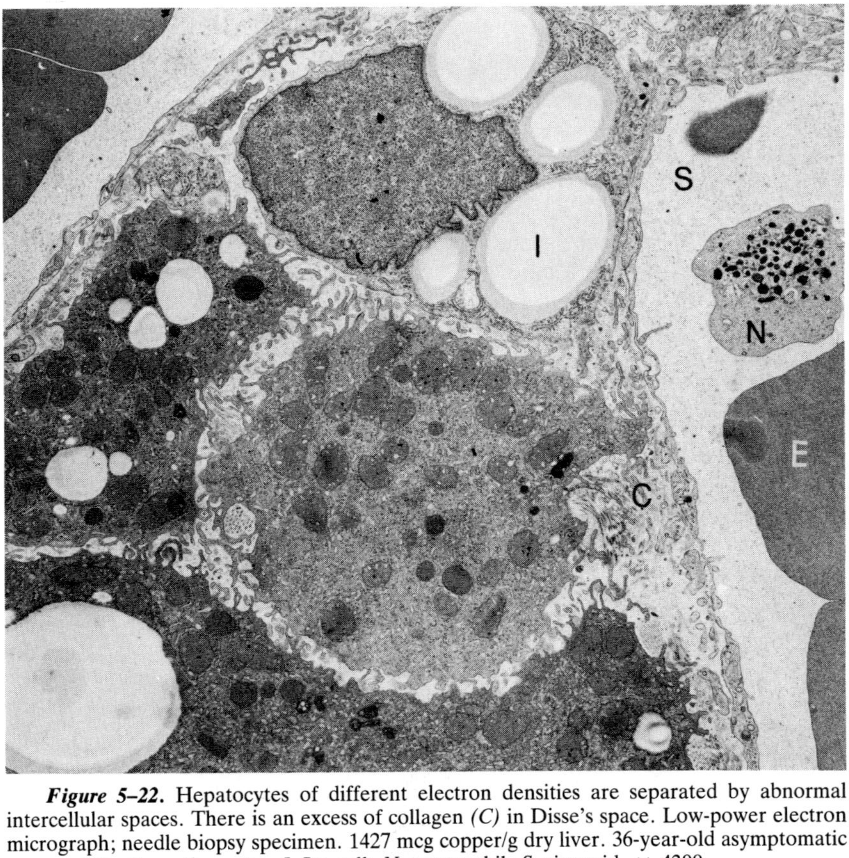

Figure 5–22. Hepatocytes of different electron densities are separated by abnormal intercellular spaces. There is an excess of collagen *(C)* in Disse's space. Low-power electron micrograph; needle biopsy specimen. 1427 mcg copper/g dry liver. 36-year-old asymptomatic woman, D2. *E*, erythrocytes; *I*, Ito cell; *N*, neutrophil; *S*, sinusoid. × 4300.

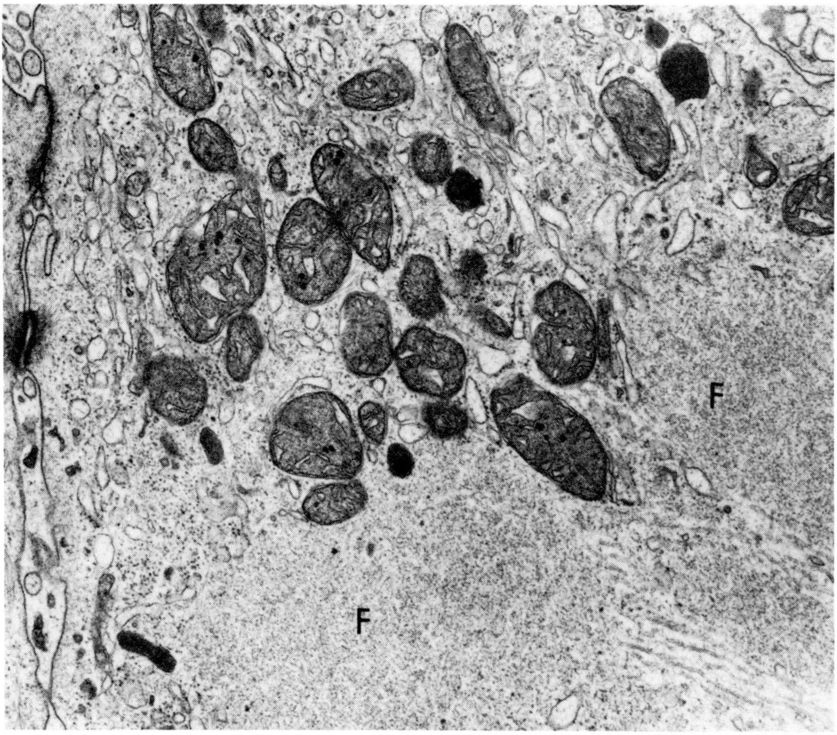

Figure 5–23. Whorls of fibrilar material *(F)* characteristic of Mallory bodies in the canalicular portion of an hepatocyte. High-power electron micrograph; needle biopsy specimen. 657 mcg copper/g dry liver. 10-year-old asymptomatic boy, S10. × 18,000.

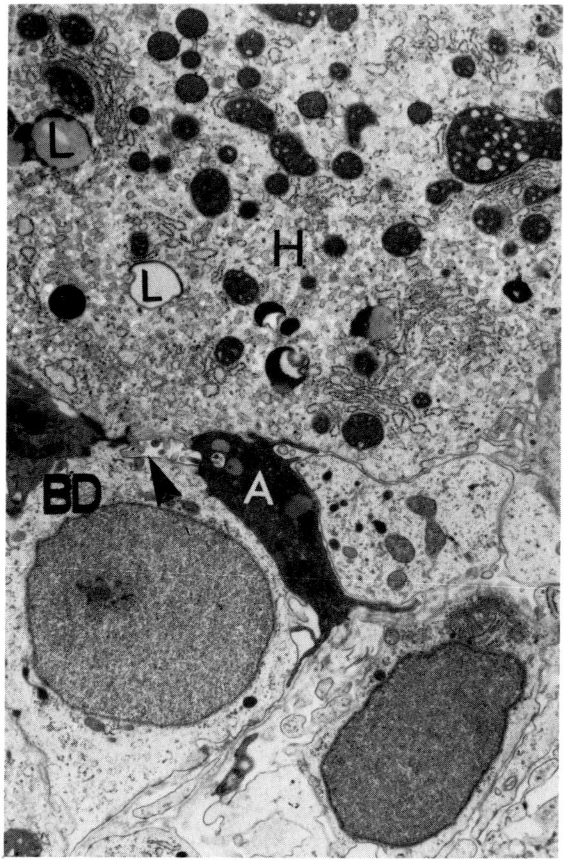

Figure 5–24. Canal of Hering (lumen indicated by arrowhead) with an hepatocyte *(H)* containing abnormal mitochondria; lipolysosomes *(L)*, membrane-bounded granules with a globular radiolucent component and an electron-dense cap that contains acid phosphatase activity; and normal *(BD)* and apoptotic *(A)* bile ductular cells. Electron micrograph; needle biopsy specimen. 1055 mcg copper/g dry tissue. 24-year-old man, E5, with neurologic and psychiatric Wilson's disease. × 3900.

Bile ductules and canals of Hering are generally, but not always, unremarkable (Figs. 5–24 and 5–25).[56, 57]

Table 5–1, summarizing the evolution of the various stages of the hepatic lesion in Wilson's disease, makes clear that the toxicity of copper to the liver is not simply a function of the mean hepatic concentration of the metal. Thus, in a normal newborn, 400 mcg copper/g dry liver—ten times the normal concentration in adults and a level diagnostic of any stage of Wilson's disease—is accompanied by normal liver structure, ultrastructure and function, presumably because the copper is sequestered in lysosomes. In a teenager with Wilson's disease, a concentration of copper only two or three times higher than that of the newborn, but diffusely distributed throughout the cytoplasm, causes pronounced cyto-

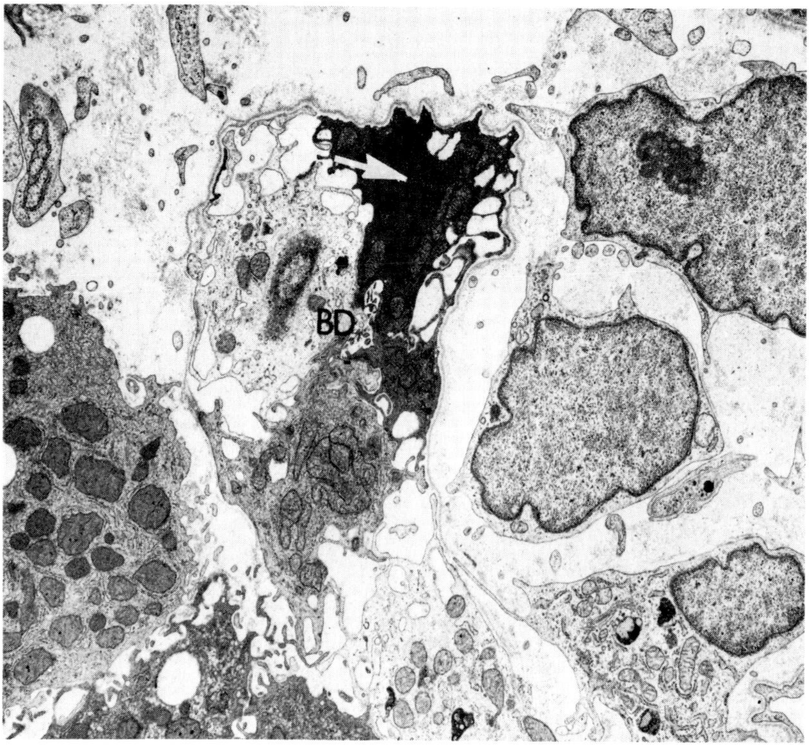

Figure 5–25. Portion of portal area with an altered bile ductule *(BD)*, with apparent apoptosis of bile ductular epithelial cells *(white arrow)* and dilated intercellular spaces, reflecting injury probably caused by the adjacent inflammatory infiltrate. Electron micrograph; needle biopsy specimen. 1158 mcg copper/g dry liver. Asymptomatic 6-year-old boy, P10. × 3500.

TABLE 5–1. Changes in the Pathologic Features Observed in Livers of Patients During the Evolution of Wilson's Disease

Feature	Early	Intermediate (Acute or Chronic Active Hepatitis)	Late
Size	Normal or enlarged	Normal, irregularly enlarged or shrunken	Normal or shrunken
Gross appearance	± Normal	Increased lobular markings	Finely or coarsely nodular
Histologic characteristics	Fatty changes, inflammation, fibrosis, glycogen nuclei	Collapse of parenchyma, portal and parenchymal fibrosis, infiltration, proliferation of bile ductules	Cirrhosis (active or quiescent)
Predominant hepatocellular abnormalities	Fatty changes, anisocytosis	Scattered fatty changes; degeneration, ballooning of hepatocytes; acidophilic bodies; Mallory bodies; nuclear unrest and enlargement	Pigment granules
Ultrastructural abnormalities	Mitochondria, peroxisomes	Not studied by electron microscopy	Excess lipofuscin
Copper concentration, mcg/g dry wt., mean ± S.D. (*n*)	983 ± 368 (*36*)	962 ± 351 (*8*)	493 ± 260 (*21*)
Copper distribution	Diffuse in cytoplasm	Diffuse in some lobules, concentrated in lysosomes in others	Concentrated in lysosomes in some lobules
Histochemical copper stains			
Specific: Rubeanic acid, rhodanine	Negative	Positive	Positive
Not specific: Timm's silver sulfide	Positive	Positive	Positive

Modified from Sternlieb, I., and Scheinberg, I. H.: Wilson's disease. In *The Liver and its Diseases*. Ed. by Schaffner, F., Sherlock, S., and Leevy, C. M., Intercontinental Medical Book Corporation, New York, 1974, pp. 328–336.

pathologic changes. Indeed, it is still an open question whether the even higher copper concentrations often present in primary biliary cirrhosis and in Indian childhood cirrhosis are toxic.[25, 58]

HEPATOCELLULAR CARCINOMA IN WILSON'S DISEASE

Hepatocellular carcinoma has developed in three (possibly four) patients[59–62] with Wilson's disease. This contrasts with the relatively common occurrence of this cancer encountered in patients with inherited hemochromatosis.[63] Three of the patients with Wilson's disease had been treated with D-penicillamine for one,[60] four[61] and 11 years.[62]

REFERENCES

1. Frerichs, F. T.: A Clinical Treatise on Diseases of the Liver, Vol. II. The New Sydenham Society, London, 1860, pp. 60–62.
2. Wilson, S. A. K.: Progressive lenticular degeneration: familial nervous disease associated with cirrhosis of liver. Brain *34*:295–509, 1911–1912.
3. Konovalov, N. V.: Hepatocerebral Dystrophy. Medgiz, Moscow, 1960.
4. Scheinberg, I. H., and Sternlieb, I.: The liver in Wilson's disease. Gastroenterology *37*:550–564, 1959.
5. Anderson, P. J., and Popper, H.: Changes in hepatic structure in Wilson's disease. Amer. J. Pathol. *36*:483–497, 1960.
6. Schaffner, F., Sternlieb, I., Barka, T., and Popper, H.: Hepatocellular changes in Wilson's disease. Histochemical and electron microscopic studies. Amer. J. Pathol. *41*:315–327, 1962.
7. Chalmers, T. C., Iber, F. L., and Uzman, L. L.: Hepatocellular degeneration (Wilson's disease) as a form of idiopathic cirrhosis. N. Engl. J. Med. *256*:235–242, 1957.
8. Shikata, T.: Liver changes in hepatocerebral disease. Acta Path. Jap. *17*:191–215, 1967.
9. Makarova, V. A., Zus, B. A., and Shulutko, B. I.: Morphology of liver cirrhosis in hepatocerebral distrophy (based on needle biopsy). Zh. Nevropatol. Psikh. (Moscow) *77*:1013–1020, 1977.
10. Odièvre, M. Vedrenne, J., Landrieu, P., and Alagille, D.: Les formes hépatiques pures de la maladie de Wilson chez l'enfant. Arch. Franç. Péd. *31*:215–222, 1974.
11. Stromeyer, F. W., and Ishak, K. G.: Histology of the liver in Wilson's disease. Amer. J. Clin. Pathol. *73*:12–24, 1980.
11a. Rojkind, M., Giambrone, M.-A., and Biempica, L.: Collagen types in normal and cirrhotic liver. Gastroenterology *76*:710–719, 1979.
11b. Sternlieb, I.: The beneficial and adverse effects of penicillamine. *In* Collagen Metabolism in the Liver. Ed. by Popper, H., and Becker, K. Stratton Intercontinental Medical Book Corp., New York, 1975, pp. 183–190.
12. Sass-Kortsak, A., and Bearn, A. G.: Hereditary disorders of copper metabolism. *In* The Metabolic Basis of Inherited Disease. Ed. by Stanbury, J. B., Wyngaarden, J. B., and Fredrickson, D. S. McGraw-Hill, New York, 1978, pp. 1098–1126.
13. Walshe, J. M.: The liver in Wilson's disease (hepatolenticular degeneration). *In* Diseases of the Liver, 5th ed. Ed. by Schiff, L., and Schiff, E. R. J. B. Lippincott, Philadelphia, 1982, pp. 1043–1059.
14. Boudin, P., Pépin, B., and Fournier, E.: Forme splénique de dégénérescence hépato-lenticulaire. Presse Méd. *65*:952–955, 1957.
15. Strickland, G. T., Chang, N. K., and Beckner, W. M.: Hypersplenism in Wilson's disease. Cut *13*:220–224, 1972.
16. Wollaegger, E. E., and Shands, H. C.: Hepatolenticular degeneration. Report of two cases with predominantly hepatogenic symptoms, one associated with Cruveilhier-Baumgarten syndrome. Arch. Int. Med. *75*:151, 1945.
17. Taylor, W. J., Jackson, E. C., and Jensen, W. N.: Wilson's disease, portal hypertension and intrahepatic vascular obstruction. N. Engl. J. Med. *260*:1160–1164, 1959.
18. Weinstein, M. P., Iannini, P. B., Stratton, C. W., and Eickhoff, T. C.: Spontaneous bacterial peritonitis. Amer. J. Med. *64*:592–598, 1978.
19. Thompson, W. G., Hyslop, P. St. G., Barr, R., and Sass-Kortsak, A.: Wilson's disease: a common liver disorder? Can. Med. Assoc. J. *117*:45–48, 1977.
20. Stein, H. L., and Watson, R. C.: Multiple intrasplenic arterial aneurysms in Wilson's disease. Amer. J. Roentgenol. Rad. Ther. Nucl. Med. *103*:441–443, 1968.

21. Duprey, R., Vallin, J., and Fabiani, F.: A propos de deux cas de maladíe de Wilson à précession hépatique chez des lithiasiques biliaires. Rev. Internat. Hépatol. *19*:233–240, 1969.
22. Rosenfield, N., Grand, R. J., Watkins, J. B., Ballantine, T. V. N., and Levey, R. H.: Cholelithiasis and Wilson's disease. J. Pediat. *92*:210–213, 1978.
23. Popper, H., and Schaffner, F.: The hepatic lesion in Wilson's disease. *In* Wilson's Disease: Some Current Concepts. Ed. by Walshe, J. M., and Cumings, J. N. Blackwell, Oxford, 1961, pp. 192–197.
23a. Arioka, I., Tanimukai, H., Nishimura, T., Nishinuma, K., and Ueda, M.: Histochemical study of hepatolenticular degeneration. Fol. Psych. Neurol. Jap. *1*:374–380, 1963.
24. Chapoy, P., Perrimond, H., Dor, A. M., Mattei, J. F., and Louchet, E.: La maladie de Wilson. Etude anatomoclinique de six observations. Sem. Hôp. Paris *55*:458–464, 1979.
25. Goldfischer, S., Popper, H., and Sternlieb, I.: The significance of variations of copper in liver disease. Amer. J. Pathol. *99*:715–730, 1980.
26. Lindquist, R. R.: Studies on the pathogenesis of hepatolenticular degeneration. II. Cytochemical methods for the localization of copper. Arch. Pathol. *87*:370–379, 1969.
27. Irons, R. D., Schenk, E. A., and Lee, J. C. K.: Cytochemical methods for copper. Arch. Pathol. Lab. Med. *101*:298–301, 1977.
28. Goldfischer, S.: Liver cell lysosomes in Wilson's disease: acid phosphatase activity by light and electron microscopy. Amer. J. Pathol. *43*:511–525, 1963.
29. Uzman, L. L.: Histochemical localization of copper with rubeanic acid. Lab. Invest. *5*:299–305, 1956.
30. Brun, A., and Voigt, G. E.: Entzündliche cerebrale Sklerose mit Nebenniereninsuffizienz. Zugleich ein Beitrag zur Histochemie von Kupferablagerungen in der Leber. Dtsch. Ztschr. Nervenhlk. *180*:654–664, 1960.
31. Goldfischer, S., and Sternlieb, I.: Changes in the distribution of hepatic copper in relation to the progression of Wilson's disease (hepatolenticular degeneration). Amer. J. Pathol. *53*:883–901, 1968.
32. Sternlieb, I., and Goldfischer, S.: Heavy metals and lysosomes. *In* Lysosomes in Biology and Pathology, Vol. 5. Ed. by Dingle, J. T., and Dean, R. T. Elsevier, New York, 1976, pp. 185–200.
33. Goldfischer, S., and Moskal, J.: Electron probe microanalysis of liver in Wilson's disease. Simultaneous assay for copper and for lead deposited by acid phosphatase activity in lysosomes. Amer. J. Pathol. *48*:305–315, 1966.
34. Sipponen, P.: Orcein positive hepatocellular material in long-standing biliary diseases. I. Histochemical characteristics. Scand. J. Gastroenterol. *11*:545–552, 1976.
34a. Johnson, G. F., Morell, A. G., Stockert, R. J., and Sternlieb, I.: Hepatic lysosomal copper protein in dogs with an inherited copper toxicosis. Hepatology *1*:243–248, 1981.
35. Goldfischer, S.: The localization of copper in the pericanalicular granules (lysosomes) of liver in Wilson's disease (hepatolenticular degeneration). Amer J. Pathol. *46*:977–983, 1965.
36. Salaspuro, M. P., Sipponen, P., and Makkonen, H.: The occurrence of orcein-positive hepatocellular material in various liver diseases. Scand. J. Gastroenterol. *11*:677–681, 1976.
37. Jain, S., Scheuer, P. J., Archer, B., Newman, S. P., and Sherlock, S.: Histological demonstration of copper and copper-associated protein in chronic liver diseases. J. Clin. Pathol. *31*:784–790, 1978.
38. Ludwig, J., McDonald, G. S. A., Dickson, E. R., Elveback, L. R., and McCall, J. T.: Copper stains and the syndrome of primary biliary cirrhosis. Arch. Pathol. Lab. Med. *103*:467–470, 1979.
39. Peters, M., Tinberg, H. M., and Govindarajan, S.: Immunocytochemical identity of hepatocellular hyalin in alcoholic and non-alcoholic liver diseases. Liver *2*:361–368, 1982.
40. Sternlieb, I.: Evolution of the hepatic lesion in Wilson's disease (hepatolenticular degeneration). *In* Progress in Liver Diseases, Vol. IV. Ed. by Popper, H., and Schaffner, F. Grune & Stratton, New York, 1972, pp. 511–525.
41. Sternlieb, I.: Mitochondrial and fatty changes in hepatocytes of patients with Wilson's disease. Gastroenterology *55*:354–367, 1968.
42. Feldmann, G., Groussard, O., and Fauvert, R.: L'ultrastructure hépatique au cours de la maladie de Wilson. Biol. Gastro-Entérol. *2*:137–160, 1969.
43. Enat. R., Lichtig, C., Segman, S., Hemli, J. A., and Barzilai, D.: Ultrastructural pathology with normal light microscopy of liver in Wilson's disease. Isr. J. Med. Sci. *15*:485–489, 1979.
44. Sternlieb, I., and Feldmann, G.: Effects of anticopper therapy on hepatocellular mitochondria in patients with Wilson's disease. Gastroenterology *71*:457–461, 1976.
45. Sternlieb, I., and Quintana, N.: The peroxisomes of human hepatocytes. Lab. Invest. *36*:140–149, 1977.
46. Angulo, A. G., Trevino, N., Perches, A., and Zavala, B. J.: Wilson's disease, an electron microscope study. Bol. Inst. Estud. Med. Biol. (Mexico) *23*:155–168, 1965.
47. Navarro, F., and Oliva, H.: Microscopia electronica del hígado en el sindromc posthepatitis y en la cirrosis de Wilson. Rev. Esp. Enferm. Apar. Dig. (Madrid) *24*:3–10, 1965.
48. Kurokawa, S., Yamawaki, T., Inagaki, T., Hayashi, H., and Okuyama, S.: Electron microscopic observation on the liver in Wilson's disease. J. Clin. Electron Microsc. *6*:99–105, 1974.
49. Makarova, V. A., and Reiskanen, A. V.: Ultrastructural changes in the liver in hepatocerebral dystrophy. Zh. Nevropatol. Psikh. (Moscow) *77*:1652–1656, 1977.
50. Lough, J., and Wiglesworth, F. W.: Wilson's disease. Comparative ultrastructure of a sibship of nine. Arch. Pathol. Lab. Med. *100*:659–663, 1976.

51. Hayashi, H., and Sternlieb, I.: Lipolysosomes in human hepatocytes. Ultrastructural and cytochemical studies of patients with Wilson's disease. Lab. Invest. *33*:1–7, 1975.
52. Sternlieb, I.: Characterization of the ultrastructure of hepatocytes in Wilson's disease. *In* Wilson's Disease. Birth Defects, Original Article Series, Vol. IV. Ed. by Bergsma, D., Scheinberg, I. H., and Sternlieb, I. The National Foundation—March of Dimes, New York, 1968, pp. 92–98.
53. Sternlieb, I., Berger, J. E., Biempica, L., Quintana, N., and Hodge, T.: Cytoplasmic crystals in human hepatocytes. Lab. Invest. *25*:503–508, 1971.
54. Biava, C., and Mukhlova-Montiel, M.: Electron microscopic observations on Councilman-like acidophilic bodies and other forms of acidophilic changes in human liver cells. Amer. J. Pathol. *46*:775–802, 1965.
55. Sternlieb, I., and Quintana, N.: Unpublished observations.
56. Sternlieb, I.: Electron microscope study of intrahepatic biliary ductules. J. Microscopie (Paris) *4*:71–80, 1965.
57. Sternlieb, I.: Functional implications of human portal and bile ductular ultrastructure. Gastroenterology *63*:321–327, 1972.
58. Epstein, O., Arborgh, B., Sagiv, M., Wroblewski. R., Scheuer, P. J., and Sherlock, S.: Is copper hepatotoxic in primary biliary cirrhosis? J. Clin. Pathol. *34*:1071–1075, 1981.
59. Lygren, T.: Hepatolenticular degeneration (Wilson's disease) and juvenile cirrhosis in the same family. Lancet *I*:275–276, 1959.
60. Vachon, A., Paliard, P., Barthe, J., Grimaud, J. A., Peyrol, Gaillard, L., and Reiss, T.: Les étapes de l'atteinte hépatique de la dégénérescence hépato-lenticulaire: lésions preécoces, hypertension portale et dégénérescence cancereuse. A propos de 4 observations. Lyon Méd. *230*:591–598, 1973.
61. Kamakura, K., Kimura, S., Igarashi, S., Fujiwara, K., Oda, T., Yoshitoshi, Y., and Shoti, S.: A case of Wilson's disease with hepatoma. J. Jap. Soc. Int. Med. *64*:232–238, 1975.
62. Terao, H., Itakura, H., Nakata, K., Kono, K., Muro, T., Furukawa, R., Kusumoto, M., Munehisa, T., Nagataki, S., Ishii, N., Koji, T., and Hirama, M.: An autopsy case of hepatocellular carcinoma in Wilson's disease. Acta Hepatol. Jap. *23*:439–445, 1982.
63. Bomford, A., and Williams, R.: Long term results of venesection therapy in idiopathic haemochromatosis. Quart. J. Med. N.S. *45*:611–623, 1976.

CHAPTER 6

NEUROPATHOLOGY

Wilson was the first to relate the neurologic manifestations of progressive hepatolenticular degeneration to pathologic changes in the basal ganglia. It has since become clear that lesions of other cerebral structures account for a number of the neurologic and psychiatric disturbances of patients with Wilson's disease.

GROSS PATHOLOGIC FINDINGS

The external surface of the intact brain is usually unremarkable.[1–4] In some cases, however, the brain is soft with marked loss of both superficial and deep white matter and with cortical shells of gyri collapsing around empty spaces.[5,6] On section, the putamina are invariably and symmetrically involved (Fig. 6–1). They are soft, have a granular, moth-

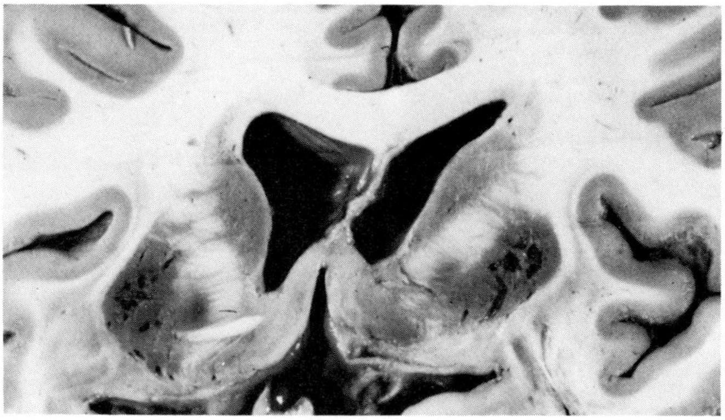

Figure 6–1. Section of brain showing cavitation of basal ganglia in patient S17 after 14 years of D-penicillamine therapy. There were no detectable neurologic abnormalities for several years before his sudden demise from complications of surgery for acutely bleeding esophageal varices. (Courtesy Dr. D. S. Horoupian.)

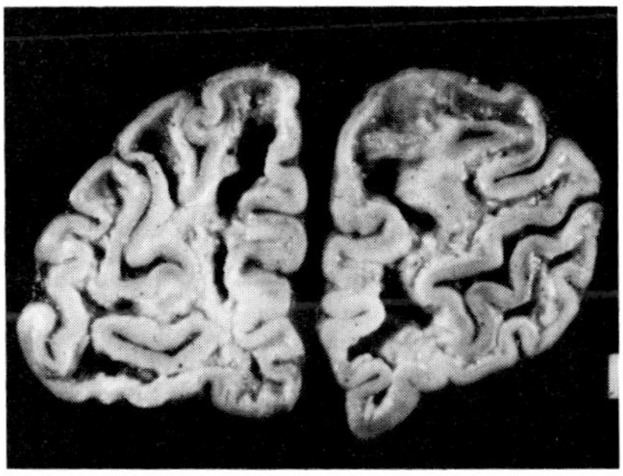

Figure 6–2. Sections of frontal lobes showing extensive cavitation of white matter with relative preservation of the cortical ribbon in the brain of patient F4, a 16-year-old boy with a five-year history of hepatic, hematologic, neurologic and psychiatric symptoms of Wilson's disease. He was in a profound coma for several months before death. (Courtesy Dr. Robert Terry.)

eaten appearance or show frank cavitation with yellowish or brownish pigmentation. Occasionally the cavitary necrosis involves the external capsule and claustrum.[1, 7] The globus pallidus is often small and discolored, but cystic degeneration is rare. The atrophy of the caudate is usually slight, and partially accounts for the flattening of its ventricular surface. The internal capsules are generally unremarkable.[1, 8] Destruction of the white matter and degeneration of the cortex are quite variable, and in perhaps 10 per cent of cases these changes may be more marked than those of the basal ganglia. Indeed, they were very severe in three reported cases[5–7] and dramatic in one case of ours (Fig. 6–2). In other instances there are no visible alterations in the deep white matter despite a cortex that is thinned to 1 to 2 mm and overlies degenerated, softened and yellowish convolutional white matter.[7]

Since the excess copper is distributed ubiquitously in the brain, it is curious that occasionally a cerebral convolution with massive disintegration may be adjacent to an apparently normal one.[7] The lateral and third ventricles are often enlarged (Fig. 6–3) because of atrophy of the basal ganglia, degeneration of the white matter or both.[1]

The external surface of the cerebellum usually appears intact, but folial atrophy of the superior vermix is sometimes observed.[1, 5–7] Frank degeneration of the white matter in the region of the dentate nucleus and spongy change have also been described.[1]

In the brain stem, central pontine myelinolysis has been reported in a number of patients with Wilson's disease[9–11] (Fig. 6–4).

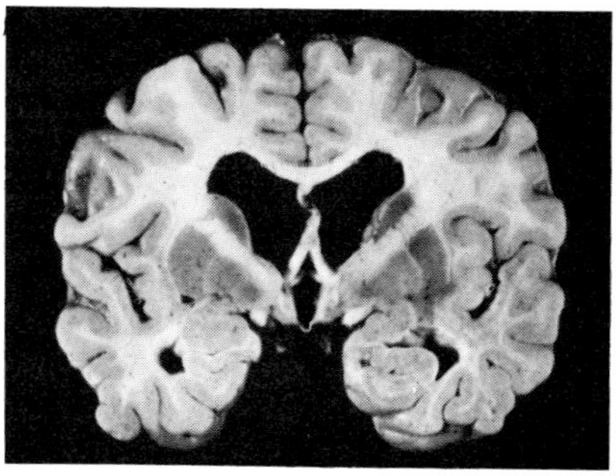

Figure 6–3. Section of brain showing symmetrical enlargement of ventricles and brown discoloration of basal ganglia in patient T7, a 47-year-old woman treated with D-penicillamine for three years. She died of sepsis following surgery for a fracture of the right hip. (Courtesy Dr. L. J. Rubinstein.)

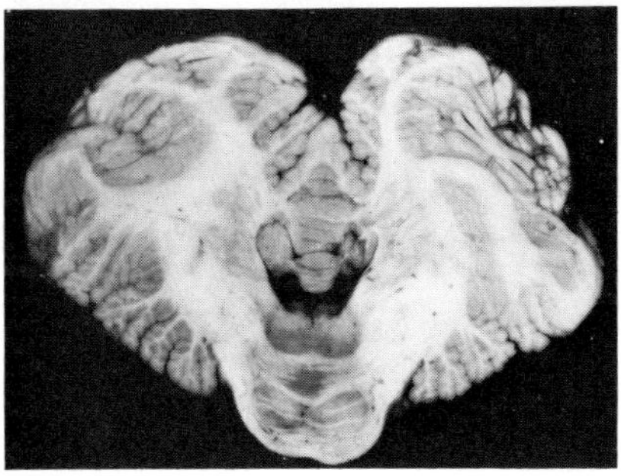

Figure 6–4. Section of cerebellum and pons showing central pontine myelinolysis in patient G1, a 47-year-old man treated with D-penicillamine for slightly less than three years (patient 1 in reference 55 of Chapter 15). (Courtesy Dr. D. S. Horoupian.)

LIGHT MICROSCOPIC FINDINGS

The striking change is a diffuse proliferation of modified protoplasmic astrocytes known as Alzheimer Type II glia[1] (Fig. 6–5). They are seen even in the absence of gross lesions in the brain, and are found in greatest concentration in the putamen, globus pallidus and caudate nucleus. Alzheimer Type II cells are characterized by a large, "naked," irregularly shaped, and usually lobulated nucleus. Some may attain 15μ in their maximal diameter. Their chromatin content is finely granular and dispersed in a clear karyoplasm. They often contain glycogen inclusions demonstrable with the PAS reaction. The cytoplasm is difficult to visualize with conventional staining techniques, but brown granules are frequently observed surrounding the nuclei. The rarer Alzheimer Type I glia are much larger, have coarse chromatin content and are frequently multinucleated.[1, 12] Neither type of Alzheimer glia is specific to Wilson's disease, and each is frequently encountered with other types of chronic liver diseases, as briefly discussed in Chapter 4.[4]

The Opalski cells generally seen in Wilson's disease are found principally in the gray matter, especially that bordering cavitary lesions.

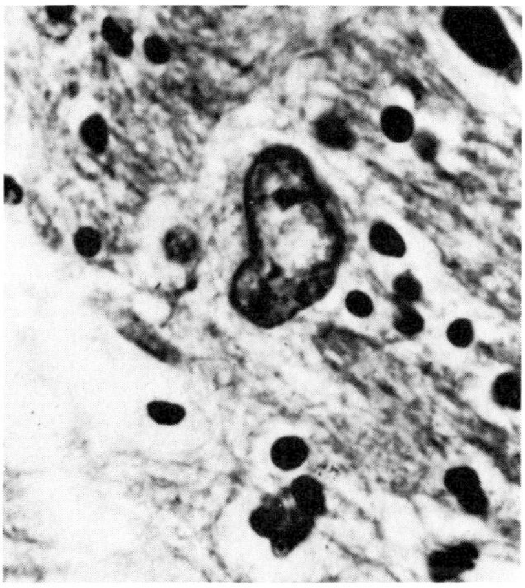

Figure 6–5. "Naked nucleus" characteristic of Alzheimer Type II glia. Histologic section of brain of patient T7. Hematoxylin-eosin. ×1200.

They are large cells with rounded contour and finely granular cytoplasm (Fig. 6–6). The nucleus is usually eccentric, pyknotic or irregularly flattened. Most of the cytoplasmic granules are PAS positive and, ultrastructurally, they are osmiophilic, resembling lysosomes. With van Gieson's stain the cytoplasm stains deep ochre.[1] Although the pathogenesis of these cells is controversial, there is a consensus that they represent degenerating astrocytes.

In the cerebral hemispheres, the deeper layers of the cortex—usually the third to fifth laminae—and the white matter are actively involved in the pathologic process.[1, 5–7] Early involvement of the cortex may be no more than capillary endothelial swelling and glial proliferation. More advanced foci show spongy change with variable degeneration or total loss of neurons. Nerve fibers with normal myelin may co-exist with others that are demyelinated. Gliosis may be diffuse, with Alzheimer Type II cells usually predominating. In the end stages there may be total dissolution of the convolutional white matter[7] with complete loss of myelinated fibers.[4]

When the cerebellum is involved, the dentate nucleus shows the most marked pathology, although the cortex or the white matter may be affected.[1, 5–7] Degeneration, or marked diminution in the number, of Purkinje cells,[6, 7] as well as proliferation of Alzheimer glia and capillaries, may be apparent.[1, 5–7] Occasionally, loss and collapse of white matter may be so severe that the dorsal and ventral laminae of the dentate are almost in contact.[1] Ultrastructural changes in Purkinje cells, including the accumulation of lipofuscin and lysosome-like granules, have been interpreted as being due to ischemia.[13]

Of the basal ganglia, the putamen is generally the most severely affected, followed by the globus pallidus, with the caudate least involved in the pathologic process. Histologic changes range from diffuse atrophy, increased numbers of astrocytes and Alzheimer cells, and degeneration of large neurones to total loss of structure, liquefaction, fissuring, spongy degeneration and cavitation. In the globus pallidus, loss of nerve fibers and demyelination may also be conspicuous. Vascular changes, ranging

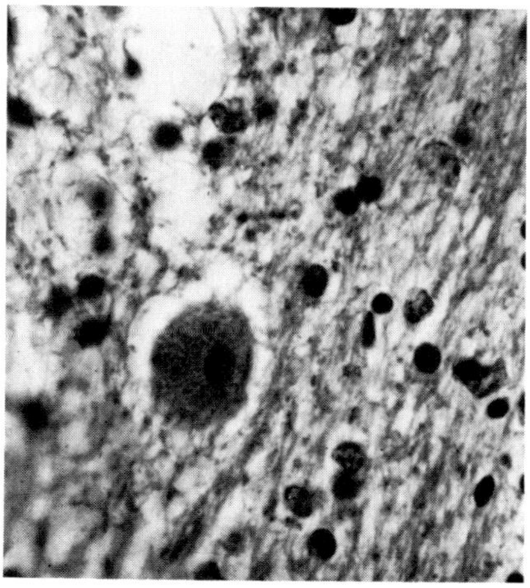

Figure 6–6. Large, rounded Opalski cell found in the gray matter of patient F4. Hematoxylin-eosin. × 700. (Courtesy Dr. Robert Terry.)

from swelling of capillary or arterial endothelium to perivascular thickening and proliferation of capillaries in areas of necrosis, associated with hemorrhagic foci, are often present in the basal ganglia. These changes have led some investigators, particularly Konovalov,[2] to suggest that the vascular lesions cause ischemic anoxia of the brain, ultimately resulting in the characteristic pathologic changes of Wilson's disease. However, it seems no less plausible to speculate that the widespread disturbances of glial cells—whether produced by ischemia or copper—may, in turn, adversely affect neurones; or that the abnormally high concentrations of copper may be the direct cause of damage to glial or nerve cells or even to blood vessels. Because patients with severe neurologic disturbances can often improve dramatically with decoppering therapy, it seems that, however caused, the neuronal pathology (short of neuronal death) is probably reversible for considerable periods of time (see Chapter 4).

In two patients with Wilson's disease, biopsy samples of brain tissue (and of peripheral nerve from one patient) have been studied by electron microscopy.[14, 15]

HISTOCHEMISTRY AND CYTOCHEMISTRY

Despite concentrations of copper that are increased ten- to fifteenfold over normal in virtually all parts of the brains of patients dying of Wilson's disease (see Table 4–1) and the certainty that the neuropathology we have just described is a result of copper toxicity, copper in patients' brain tissue is often not histochemically stainable with rubeanic acid or rhodanine,[16, 17] although more sensitive stains (e.g., Timm's silver sulfide) can demonstrate the metal. We have pointed out in Chapter 5 that an analogous situation is not uncommonly found in the livers of Wilson's disease patients, where similarly elevated concentrations of copper may be histochemically detectable only with such sensitive stains during stages of the disease when the excess hepatocytic copper is diffusely distributed.

Quantitative measurements of brain copper concentrations (see Table 4–1) show that there is no correlation of tissue copper excess with the sites of pathology and that the brains of treated patients have only moderately lower concentrations of copper than those of untreated patients. Most of the excess brain copper in patients with Wilson's disease is bound to a number of proteins, none of which appears to differ from the proteins of normal brain except in their binding of copper.[18]

REFERENCES

1. Schulman, S.: Wilson's disease. *In* Pathology of the Nervous System, Vol. 1. Ed. by Minckler, J. McGraw-Hill, New York, 1968, pp. 1139–1151.
2. Konovalov, N. V.: Hepatocerebral Dystrophy. Medgiz, Moscow, 1960.
3. Boudin, G., and Pépin, B.: Dégénérescence hépatolenticulaire, Masson, Paris, 1959.
4. Shiraki, H.: Comparative neuropathologic study of Wilson's disease and other types of hepatocerebral disease. *In* Wilson's Disease. Birth Defects, Original Article Series, Vol. IV. Ed. by Bergsma, D., Scheinberg, I. H., and Sternlieb, I. The National Foundation—March of Dimes, New York, 1968, pp. 64–73.
5. Schulman, S., and Barbeau, A.: Wilson's disease: a case with almost total loss of cerebral white matter. J. Neuropath. Exp. Neur. *22*:105–119, 1963.

6. Ishino, H., Takashi, M., Hayashi, Y., Saito, A., and Otsuki, S.: A case of Wilson's disease with enormous cavity formation of cerebral white matter. Neurology *22*:905–909, 1972.
7. Richter, R.: The pallial component in hepato-lenticular degeneration. J. Neuropath. Exp. Neur. *7*:1–18, 1948.
8. Martin, J. P.: Wilson's disease. *In* Handbook of Clinical Neurology. Vol. 6. Ed. by Vinken, P. J., and Bruyn, G. W., John Wiley & Sons, New York, 1968, pp. 267–278.
9. Popoff, N., Budzilovicch, G., Goodgold, A., and Feigin, I.: Hepatocerebral degeneration. Its occurrence in the presence and in the absence of abnormal copper metabolism. Neurology *15*:919–930, 1965.
10. Castan, P.: La myélinolyse centrale dans la dégénérescence hépato-lenticulaire. Essai sur sa signification. Rev. Neur. (Paris) *117*:391–409, 1967.
11. Seitelberger, F.: Zentrale pontine Myelinolyse. Schweiz. Arch. Neurol. Neurochir. u. Psych. *112*:285–297, 1973.
12. Tarnowska-Dziduszko, E., and Wald, I.: Study on glial changes in hepato-lenticular degeneration. Polish Med. J. *10*:743–749, 1971.
13. Ohta, K., Okamoto, Y., Honda, O., Ogata, M., and Takahashi, K.: Electron microscopic observations on the cerebellar cortex of a case of Wilson's disease. Psych. Neurol. Japon. *72*:157–169 (English abstract, pp. 224–225), 1970.
14. Ohta, K., Okamoto, Y., and Honda, O.: Electron microscopic observations on the cerebrum of a case of Wilson's disease. Psych. Neurol. Japon. *71*:385–406 (English abstract, p. 432), 1969.
15. Anzil, A. P., Herrlinger, H., Blinzinger, K., and Heldrich, A.: Ultrastructure of brain and nerve biopsy tissue in Wilson disease. Arch. Neurol. *31*:94–100, 1974.
16. Uzman, L. L.: Histochemical localization of copper with rubeanic acid. Lab. Invest. *5*:299–305, 1956.
17. Levina, G. Ia.: Localization of copper in the brain in hepato-cerebral dystrophy. Zh. Nevropat. Psikh. *67*:990–993, 1967.
18. Porter, H.: Copper proteins in brain and liver in normal subjects and in cases of Wilson's disease. *In* Wilson's Disease, Birth Defects, Original Article Series, Vol. IV. Ed. by Bergsma, D., Scheinberg, I. H., and Sternlieb, I. The National Foundation—March of Dimes, New York, 1968, pp. 23–28.

CHAPTER 7

THE LIVER: CLINICAL ASPECTS

In Wilson's disease the liver is both the site of the fundamental genetic defect in copper metabolism and the primary target of copper toxicity, as is apparent in Chapter 4. Clinically overt manifestations of hepatic copper toxicosis have never been seen before five years of age.[1–12] During this asymptomatic period, which may extend well into adult life, some or all of the following are almost always present: hepatomegaly, splenomegaly, scattered spider angiomas (particularly on the dorsum of the hand), or moderate elevations of serum aminotransferase levels. If the cause of any of these abnormalities is not certain, in a young person, the physician should carry out corneal slit-lamp examination, determination of the serum ceruloplasmin concentration, and hepatic biopsy—all generally necessary to confirm or exclude the diagnosis. If the diagnosis is Wilson's disease, unless specific decoppering treatment is instituted before the hepatic pathology becomes clinically manifest, liver disease eventually evolves in one of four discrete ways.

1. Acute hepatitis. An acute, self-limited illness, often characterized by jaundice, lassitude, and anorexia appears to have been the first clinical manifestation of Wilson's disease in 24 per cent of our patients with this disorder. Subsiding spontaneously, the illness may be ascribed falsely to a viral infection or, when splenomegaly is detected, to infectious mononucleosis.[5] Hepatitis associated with a transient hemolytic anemia, unconjugated hyperbilirubinemia or hypouricemia should suggest that Wilson's disease may be the underlying disorder. Recovery is usually so complete that the episode itself may be forgotten, or recalled, years later, only under direct questioning. In a number of instances patients of this sort are told, at the time of their hepatitis, that they have had infectious mononucleosis.

A 17-year-old daughter, J1, of unrelated Jewish parents complained of postprandial abdominal distension and fatigue, cramps of legs and toes, and depression. When she became almost constantly

sleepy and deeply icteric and exhibited slight hepatosplenomegaly, she was thought to have infectious mononucleosis. Hemoglobin was 7.2 g/dl; hematocrit, 21%; reticulocyte count, 6.7%; leukocytes, 16,000; glucose, 84 mg/dl; blood urea nitrogen, 9 mg/dl; total serum bilirubin, 17 mg/dl; total serum proteins, 6.6 g/dl with an albumin of 3.5 g/dl; SGOT, 130 mU/ml; alkaline phosphatase, 29 mU/ml; inorganic serum phosphorus, 0.8 mg/dl; and serum uric acid, 1.5 mg/dl. Her hemolytic anemia was Coombs negative.

Transfusion of four units of blood was followed, within four days, by a fall in the serum bilirubin to 2.4 mg/dl. She continued to improve rapidly and was discharged within one week with no further investigation of the cause of her illness, hypophosphatemia or hypouricemia.

In an older sister, J3, there soon developed severe and irreversible neurologic manifestations that were correctly recognized as due to Wilson's disease. J1 was then also shown to have the disorder when re-investigation revealed Kayser-Fleischer rings, hypoceruloplasminemia, and hypercupriuria.

2. Fulminant hepatitis. In adolescent patients—and a very few older ones—the course of the disease may be so severe that the initial acute hepatitis progresses within a few weeks to severe hepatic insufficiency, deep jaundice, encephalopathy, edema, ascites, severe clotting abnormalities (occasionally with intravascular coagulation), terminal renal insufficiency and, almost always, death.[13–23a] Without a history of hepatic or neurologic disease in the family (and occasionally *with* it), the physician almost invariably considers the illness to be an acquired episode of viral or toxic etiology, since the symptomatology and findings are not specific. (The physician may even be misled into minimizing the seriousness of the illness, since the submassive hepatic necrosis may cause, for unknown reasons, only minimally elevated aminotransferase levels and, even in adolescents, normal adult alkaline phosphatase concentrations.) This clinical picture, if accompanied by a profound, Coombs-negative, hemolytic anemia, is more likely to be Wilson's disease than any other disorder. Unfortunately, the diagnostic importance and specificity of hemolysis accompanied by marked hypercupremia and hypercupriuria are rarely recognized. Unless the physician thinks of Wilson's disease, obtains the pertinent laboratory data, and asks an ophthalmologist to ascertain whether Kayser-Fleischer rings are present, the diagnosis will rarely be made except by an alert pathologist at autopsy.

A healthy 20-year-old college student, A1, whose past history was noteworthy only because of irregular menses, was seen by a physician because of malaise, anorexia, nausea, fatigue, and a spontaneous seven-pound weight loss. She had not taken any drugs, nor had she been exposed to toxic chemicals. Physical examination was unremarkable. Bilirubin was 1.8 mg/dl; SGOT, 75 mU/ml; alkaline phosphatase, normal; hemoglobin, 13 g/dl; leukocyte count, normal; but platelets were 24,000. Despite a negative heterophile test, a diagnosis of infectious mononucleosis was made. The abnormalities in her blood were significantly worse a week after the initial values were taken. Three weeks after the latter, bilirubin was 18 mg/dl; SGOT, 375 mU/ml; leukocyte count, 25,000; and the hemoglobin had dropped to 8 g/dl. Wilson's disease was suspected because of a decreased serum uric acid level, and the diagnosis was confirmed

when Kayser-Fleischer rings were seen. By then she had become obtunded, with asterixis, anuria and deep jaundice reflecting a serum bilirubin of 59 mg/dl. Sudden hypotension and cardiac arrest occurred less than one month after the onset of her acute illness.

A very similar course of events can occur in patients with Wilson's disease who have been treated effectively—and who may even have been maintained in the asymptomatic state—but who have discontinued penicillamine therapy for as little as nine months. Their deaths are usually the paradoxical results of their successful therapy, since they eventually come to believe that their continued good health is unrelated to the penicillamine they have been taking.

An 11-year-old boy, M1, was in excellent health when, following the diagnosis of Wilson's disease in his older brother, he was found to have faint bilateral Kayser-Fleischer crescents, no detectable serum ceruloplasmin, a total serum copper of 9 mcg/dl with histopathologic changes in the liver characteristic of Wilson's disease and a copper concentration of 956 mcg/g dry liver. Penicillamine treatment was promptly instituted and continued for the following 12 years, during which time he remained asymptomatic.

He then stopped taking penicillamine, and did not return to his physician but apparently remained in good health for 6 years. When he was 29, he complained of tiredness, and his local physician, noting rapidly deepening jaundice, admitted him to the hospital, where his serum bilirubin was 15 mg/dl; total serum proteins, 6.5 g/dl; albumin, 2.7 g/dl; but both alkaline phosphatase and SGOT were normal. His condition steadily deteriorated, with the development of sepsis and gastrointestinal hemorrhage. He died less than a month later.

3. Chronic active hepatitis. Since our first report in 1972,[24] a number of papers[12, 25–30] have confirmed that Wilson's disease may present, particularly in young patients, with a clinical picture indistinguishable from that of chronic active hepatitis of viral etiology: the febrile or afebrile development—insidious or sudden—of malaise, fatigue and anorexia with vague or localized abdominal complaints. Any combination of polyarthralgias, amenorrhea, delayed puberty, gynecomastia, bruisability, low-grade jaundice, edema or ascites may also be seen. The liver may be slightly enlarged, firm and nodular, and splenomegaly is usually present. The laboratory findings of persistent hypoalbuminemia, aminotransferase and serum gamma globulin elevations and the histologic appearance of the hepatic biopsy sample will usually, and understandably, lead to a diagnosis of viral or drug-induced chronic active hepatitis (see Chapter 5). Unfortunately, even if Wilson's disease *is* suspected, the physician may be erroneously convinced that the diagnosis is not tenable in the absence of Kayser-Fleischer rings or in the presence of a serum ceruloplasmin concentration made temporarily normal by the stimulus of the inflammatory process[31, 32] (see Chapter 3). If a viral etiology cannot be established, it is essential, therefore, that a quantitative hepatic copper concentration be determined on an hepatic biopsy sample, or, if there is a contraindication to liver biopsy, that a radiocopper loading test be carried out to resolve the issue if rings are absent and the ceruloplasmin is normal.[33] If the correct diagnosis of Wilson's disease is *not* made, the patient is doomed; if it *is* made, and penicillamine given, the results are almost certain to be gratifying.

In 1962, his medical history having previously been uneventful, lymphadenopathy, epigastric pain, fever and hepatosplenomegaly developed in this 20-year-old medical student, S1. A diagnosis of infectious mononucleosis was made, although heterophile agglutination was positive only in a titer of 1:14. An SGPT of 219 Karmen units/ml was reported. He recovered completely, though splenomegaly persisted.

Six years later, when he passed a calcium oxalate stone, with colic, transaminase values were normal. Within a month of this episode, malaise, right upper quadrant soreness, slight jaundice and transaminase values of 800 to 1000 IU led to hospitalization. Although mildly febrile and obtunded, his only symptoms were diarrhea and urinary frequency. He convalesced slowly, with transaminase elevations of about 60 IU persisting.

Because of continued mild malaise, slight elevation in alkaline phosphatase, and the presence of Hepatitis B_S antibody in his serum, a liver biopsy was performed in late 1969. The copper concentration of the sample was not determined, and since the histologic appearance of the sample was interpreted as "resolving chronic active hepatitis" (Fig. 3 in reference 24), no treatment was prescribed. Symptoms and laboratory findings were essentially unchanged throughout the ensuing year.

In November 1970, because of mild conjunctivitis, he consulted an ophthalmologist, who discovered bilateral Kayser-Fleischer rings. Deficiency of serum ceruloplasmin (15.1 mg/dl) and an elevated urinary 24-hour urinary copper excretion (390 mcg) confirmed the diagnosis of Wilson's disease.

4. Cirrhosis. We have seen the cirrhosis of Wilson's disease kill a child of 8 (G8), and remain clinically latent until 51 (G9). Cirrhosis is present in all patients with neurologic disturbances, but it is not always silent throughout their lives, as Wilson believed.[2, 34, 35] Indeed, of a large series of patients in the German Democratic Republic[36] the illness of nearly half *began* with signs and symptoms of cirrhosis: fatigue, anorexia, abdominal pain, weight loss; edema, ascites, anasarca; jaundice; epistaxis (and other bleeding phenomena); primary or secondary amenorrhea; infertility; miscarriages (perhaps attributable to intrauterine free copper); gynecomastia, delayed male puberty; spider angiomas; susceptibility to bacteremia and bacterial peritonitis; encephalopathy with asterixis, confusion, obtunded sensorium, and coma; or terminal hepatorenal syndrome.

Secondary to portal hypertension[37, 38] there may be marked splenomegaly, hypersplenism,[39] splenic infarction or esophageal variceal bleeding.[40]

Since all of these manifestations can occur in cirrhosis of any etiology, patients with Wilsonian cirrhosis and no neurologic abnormalities are, tragically, all too frequently misdiagnosed as having juvenile, cryptogenic or alcoholic cirrhosis; Banti's syndrome; or idiopathic thrombocytopenic purpura.

Physical examination may show the liver to be normal in size, shrunken, or, rarely, enlarged, with an edge that is firm and nodular. The splenic tip may be barely palpable, or the organ may be enlarged to fill the entire left side of the abdomen. Spider angiomas are commonly seen in younger patients; superficial collateral venous channels much less frequently. Esophageal or gastric varices may be demonstrable by x-ray or endoscopy. The few wedged hepatic vein pressures that have been measured have usually been found to be normal, indicating that the portal hypertension is of the presinusoidal type,[37] although this is not invariably so.[41]

The commonest biochemical disturbance is of moderate elevations of aminotransferase levels, but any combination of abnormalities in the serum concentrations of albumin, gamma globulin, prothrombin, alkaline phosphatase and bilirubin may be seen, depending on the degree of hepatic decompensation. Bromsulphalein clearance is normal often enough so that this test is of little diagnostic or prognostic value.[42] Clearance of glycine conjugates of cholic acid, although reported in only one study, may provide a more sensitive indicator of hepatic dysfunction.[43] Ultrasound or radionuclide studies of the liver and spleen are nonspecific.

Bleeding and bruising are not uncommon, although they were the initial complaints of only two of 151 patients; they may be due to defective hepatic synthesis of fibrinogen, Factors II, V, VII, X or prothrombin[44, 45] or to hypersplenic thrombocytopenic purpura.[39, 46] Functionally defective platelets have been described,[47, 48] and shortened red cell survival[39, 49] (similar to that seen in other forms of cirrhosis) may be responsible for the apparently increased incidence of bilirubin-containing gallstones in Wilson's disease.[50]

Unless esophageal variceal bleeding,[40] sepsis, bacterial peritonitis[51] or submassive necrosis with hemolysis is either quickly fatal or initiates progressive hepatic decompensation, Wilsonian cirrhosis is remarkably well tolerated in the majority of patients. With decompensation, however, the electrolyte imbalance, uncontrollable bleeding, renal insufficiency and hepatic coma of advanced cirrhosis are all too often so poorly responsive to diuretics, blood or albumin infusions, dialysis,[19] and treatment of encephalopathy that a fatal outcome can be prevented only by a successful liver transplant.[52]

P1, the youngest of three sons of unrelated parents, began to lie and erupt in bursts of anger at about 11 years. At 15 he curtailed his physical activities because of fatigue. A physician, consulted because of abdominal pain, discovered a finely nodular, firm, enlarged liver, marked splenomegaly, ascites, scleral icterus, spider angiomas and bilateral Kayser-Fleischer rings. Total bilirubin was 5.7 mg/dl; total serum proteins, 7 g/dl; serum albumin, 2.4 g/dl; SGOT, 325 mU/ml; SGPT, 182 mU/ml; alkaline phosphatase, 127 IU; prothrombin time, 18/11 seconds; serum uric acid, 1.6 mg/dl; and serum phosphorus, 1.8 mg/dl. Serum ceruloplasmin was 9 mg/dl; serum copper, 70 mcg/dl; and 24-hour urinary copper, 1750 mcg. Tests for serologic markers of hepatitis were all negative.

A therapeutic regimen that included penicillamine, restriction of dietary copper and sodium, spironolactone, furosemide and multivitamins was instituted. Despite it, ascites, deepening jaundice, Klebsiella and enterococcal septicemia, anemia, clotting abnormalities,

renal insufficiency and hepatic encephalopathy culminated in an episode of massive esophageal variceal bleeding and death about six months after his first symptoms of liver disease (see Fig. 5–1,*B*).

At 13, irritability, easy bruisability, epistaxes, and slurred speech were noted in M2, the daughter of unrelated parents. At 16, tonsillectomy was performed because of her dysarthria, and was complicated by excessive postoperative bleeding. Shortly thereafter, abdominal distension and massive bodily edema appeared. Wilson's disease, then suspected because of the dysarthria, liver disease and amenorrhea, was confirmed by the demonstration of Kayser-Fleischer rings; serum ceruloplasmin, 8.9 mg/dl; serum copper, 46 mcg/dl; and 24-hour urinary copper, 170 mcg. Total serum proteins were 7.5 g/dl; serum albumin, 2.8 g/dl; SGOT, 25 mU/ml; prothrombin time 17.4/11 seconds; serum phosphorus, 3.6 mg/dl; and uric acid 3.6 mg/dl.

She was hospitalized for eight months on a regimen including penicillamine (1 to 3 g/day), a diet low in copper and salt, spironolactone, thiazide diuretics, pyridoxine, multivitamins, and two courses of BAL. She slowly improved, with the loss of 50 pounds (all edema) and an increase in her serum albumin to 54 per cent of total serum proteins, and diuretics and salt restriction were discontinued.

Although secondary sex characteristics developed and she became pregnant twice, she never menstruated. She lived and worked essentially normally, with penicillamine treatment continued, for seven years, when she died following a third episode of esophageal variceal bleeding.

Three unusual features of Wilsonian liver disease require comment.

First, Wilsonian cirrhosis rarely evolves into hepatocellular carcinoma, in contrast to the higher incidence of the latter in the more common forms of cirrhosis. Only four instances of this association have been reported[53–56] of which three have been confirmed.[54–56] Since hepatocellular carcinoma is also known to be an unusual development in patients with primary biliary cirrhosis, it is possible that abnormally elevated concentrations of copper, which are pathognomonic of both of these forms of cirrhosis and which have been shown to suppress the incorporation of ^{3}H-thymidine into rat liver DNA,[57] may act to prevent carcinogenesis in the liver.

Second, cholelithiasis, which occurs in children and adults with Wilson's disease, may account for some episodes of abdominal pain.[50]

Third, a number of patients with Wilson's disease exhibit a slight, but definite, elevation in the plasma concentration of unconjugated bilirubin, as first reported by Black and Billing.[58] This may represent coincidental occurrences of both Wilson's disease and Gilbert's syndrome in these patients, or it may be an effect of copper on UDP glucuronyl transferase activity.

REFERENCES

1. Kehrer, F.: Aetiologie und Nosologie der Pseudosklerose Westphal-Wilson. Z. Ges. Neurol. Psychiatr. *129*:448–542, 1930.
2. Konovalov, N. V.: Hepatocerebral Dystrophy. Medgiz, Moscow, 1960.
3. Cartwright, G. E., Hodges, R. E., Gubler, C. J., Mahoney, J. P., Daum, K., Wintrobe, M. M.,

and Bean, W. B.: Studies on copper metabolism XIII. Hepatolenticular degeneration. J. Clin. Invest. *33*:1487–1501, 1954.
4. Walshe, J. M.: Wilson's disease (hepatolenticular degeneration). *In* Handbook of Clinical Neurology. Ed. by Vinken, P. J., and Bruyn, G. W. Elsevier, New York, 1976, pp. 379–414.
5. Silverberg, M., and Gellis, S. S.: The liver in juvenile Wilson's disease. Pediatrics *30*:402–413, 1962.
6. Strickland, G. T., Frommer, D., Leu, M. L., Pollard, R., Sherlock, S., and Cumings, J. N.: Wilson's disease in the United Kingdom and Taiwan. Quart. J. Med. *62*:619–638, 1973.
7. Sass-Kortsak, A., and Bearn, A. G.: Hereditary disorders of copper metabolism. *In* The Metabolic Basis of Inherited Disease. Ed. by Stanbury, J. B., Wyngaarden, J. B., and Fredickson, D. S. McGraw-Hill, New York, 1978, pp. 1098–1126.
8. Arima, M., Komiya, K., Kamoshita, S., and Mukai, N.: Clinical and pathological characteristics in Wilson's disease under ten years of age. Paediatria Univ. Tokyo 9:17–22, 1963.
9. Sternlieb, I., and Scheinberg, I. H.: Wilson's disease. *In* Liver and Biliary Disease. A Pathophysiological Approach. Ed. by Wright, R., Alberti, K. G. M. M., Karran, S., and Milward-Sadler, G. H. W. B. Saunders, Philadelphia, 1979, pp. 774–787.
10. Slovis, T. L., Dubois, R. S., Rodgerson, D. O., and Silverman, A.: The varied manifestations of Wilson's disease. J. Pediatr. *78*:578–584, 1971.
11. Bachmann, H., Willgerodth, H., Ruchholtz, U., Biesold, D., and Lössner, J.: Über die abdominale Verlaufsform der Wilsonschen Erkrankung und ihre Bedeutung für Früherkennung und Familienberatung. Dtsch. Gesundh. Wesen *35*:1103–1107, 1980.
12. Stromeyer, F. W., and Ishak, K. G.: Histology of the liver in Wilson's disease. Amer. J. Clin. Pathol. *73*:12–24, 1980.
13. McIntyre, N., Clink, H. M., Levi, A. J., Cumings, J. N., and Sherlock, S.: Hemolytic anemia in Wilson's disease. N. Engl. J. Med. *276*:439–444, 1967.
14. Deiss, A., Lee, G. R., and Cartwright, G. E.: Hemolytic anemia in Wilson's disease. Ann. Intern. Med. *73*:413–418, 1970.
15. Passwell, J., Cohen, B. E., Ben Bassat, I., Ramot, B., Shchory, M., and Lavi, U.: Hemolysis in Wilson's disease. The role of glucose-6-phosphate dehydrogenase. Isr. J. Med. Sci. *6*:549–554, 1970.
16. Tönz, O., Furrer, H. U., and Bangerter, U.: Kupferinduzierte Hämolyse bei Morbus Wilson. Schweiz. Med. Wschr. *101*:1800–1802, 1971.
17. Willms, B., Blume, K. G., and Lohr, G. W.: Hämolytische Anämie bei Morbus Wilson (Hepatolentikulare Degeneration). Klin. Wschr. *50*:995–1002, 1972.
18. Roche-Sicot, J., and Benhamou, J.-P.: Acute intravascular hemolysis and acute liver failure associated as a first manifestation of Wilson's disease. Ann. Intern. Med. *86*:301–303, 1977.
19. Hamlyn, A. N., Gollan, J. L., Douglas, A. P., and Sherlock, S.: Fulminant Wilson's disease with haemolysis and renal failure: copper studies and assessment of dialysis regimens. Brit. Med. J. *2*:660–663, 1977.
20. Storck, D., Bareiss, P., Jesel, B., and Warter, J.: L'ictère grave hémolytique de la maladie de Wilson. Sem. Hôp. Paris, *52*:2407–2412, 1976.
21. Adler, R., Mahnovski, V., Heuser, E. T., Presser, D. H., and Robinson, R. G.: Fulminant hepatitis: a presentation of Wilson's disease. Amer. J. Dis. Child. *131*:870–872, 1977.
22. Doering, E. J., III, Savage, R. A., and Dittmer, T. E.: Hemolysis, coagulation defects, and fulminant hepatic failure as a presentation of Wilson's disease. Amer. J. Dis. Child. *133*:440–441, 1979.
23. Forman, S. J., Kumar, K. S., Redeker, A. G., and Hochstein, P.: Hemolytic anemia in Wilson's disease: clinical findings and biochemical mechanisms. Amer. J. Hematol. *9*:269–275, 1980.
23a. McCullough, A. J., Fleming, C. R., Thistle, J. L., Baldus, W. P., Ludwig, J., McCall, J. T., and Dickson, E. R.: Diagnosis of Wilson's disease presenting as fulminant hepatic failure. Gastroenterology *84*:161–167, 1983.
24. Sternlieb, I., and Scheinberg, I. H.: Chronic hepatitis as a first manifestation of Wilson's disease. Ann. Intern. Med. *76*:59–64, 1972.
25. Odièvre, M., Vedrenne, J., Landrieu, P., and Alagille, D.: Les formes hépatiques "pures" de la maladie de Wilson chez l'enfant Arch. Franç. Péd. *31*:215–222, 1974.
26. Johnson, R. C., Deford, J. W., and Gebhart, R. J.: Chronic active hepatitis and cirrhosis in Wilson's disease. South Med. J. *70*:753–754, 1977.
27. Izquierdo, A. N., Carton, J. A., Ubeda, I., Zaboy, J. M., and DeVillalobos, E.: Hepatitis cronica activa como unica manifestacion de la enfermedad de Wilson. Rev. Clin. Esp. *151*:293–295, 1978.
28. Scott, J., Gollan, J. L., Samourian, S., and Sherlock, S.: Wilson's disease, presenting as chronic active hepatitis. Gastroenterology *74*:645–651, 1978.
29. Perman, J. A., Werlin, S. L., Grand, R. J., and Watkins, J. B.: Laboratory measures of copper metabolism in the differentiation of chronic active hepatitis and Wilson's disease in children. J. Pediatr. *94*:564–568, 1979.
30. Spechler, S. J., and Koff, R. S.: Wilson's disease: diagnostic difficulties in the patient with chronic hepatitis and hypoceruloplasminemia. Gastroenterology *78*:803–806, 1980.
31. Scheinberg, I. H., and Sternlieb, I.: Wilson's disease and the concentration of caeruloplasmin in serum. Lancet, *I*:1420–1421, 1963.
32. Walshe, J. M.: Wilson's disease and chronic active hepatitis. Lancet *I*:605–606, 1977.
33. Sternlieb, I., and Scheinberg, I. H.: The role of radiocopper in the diagnosis of Wilson's disease. Gastroenterology *77*:138–142, 1979.

34. Barnes, S., and Hurst, E. W.: Hepato-lenticular degeneration. Brain *48*:279–333, 1925.
35. Boudin, G., and Pépin, B.: Dégénérescence Hépatolenticulaire. Masson, Paris, 1959.
36. Lössner, J., Bachmann, H., Biesold, D., Ruchholtz, U., and Storch, W.: Untersuchungen zur Wilsonshen Erkrankung in der DDR. Z. Ges. Inn. Med. *35*:136–140, 1980.
37. Taylor, W. J., Jackson, E. C., and Jensen, W. N.: Wilson's disease, portal hypertension and extrahepatic vascular obstruction. N. Engl. J. Med. *260*:1160–1164, 1959.
38. Seidlová, V., and Kuba, J.: Der portale Kreislauf bei langfristig mit D-Penicillamin benhandelten Leberparenchymschäden, verursacht durch einen Morbus Wilson, Dtsch. Z. Verdau u. Stoffwechselkr. *35*:17–23, 1975.
39. Strickland, G. T., Chang, N. K., and Beckner, W. M.: Hypersplenism in Wilson's disease. Gut *13*:220–224, 1972.
40. Sternlieb, I., Scheinberg, I. H., and Walshe, J. M.: Bleeding oesophageal varices in patients with Wilson's disease. Lancet *1*:638–641, 1970.
41. Takasaki, H., Murata, S., Saiki, K., Kosaka, Y., Ikeda, N., and Matuda, Y.: A case report of Wilson's disease. Gastroenterol. Jap. *1*:54, 1966.
42. Schoenfield, L. J., Onstad, G. R., and Goldstein, N. P.: Normal sulfobromophthalein retention in established liver disease. Amer. J. Digest. Dis. *15*:337–342, 1970.
43. Cowen, A. E., Korman, M. G., Hofmann, A. F., and Goldstein, N. P.: Biliary bile acid composition in Wilson's disease. Mayo Clin. Proc. *50*:229–233, 1975.
44. Prochazká, J., and Hauftová, D.: Changes of some clotting factors in hepatolenticular degeneration (Wilson's disease). Gastroenterologia *104*:325–334, 1964.
45. Fischer, H., Hayek, H., Schnack, H., Schenck, W., Bauer, B., and Kunzer, W.: Veränderungen der Blutgerinnung bei Morbus Wilson. Dtsch. Med. Wschr. *93*:1229–1232, 1968.
46. Hoagland, H. C., and Goldstein, N.: Hematologic (cytopenic) manifestations of Wilson's disease (hepatolenticular degeneration). Mayo Clin. Proc. *53*:498–500, 1978.
47. Owen, C. A., Goldstein, N. P., and Bowie, E. J. W.: Platelet function and coagulation in patients with Wilson's disease. Arch. Int. Med. *136*:148–152, 1976.
48. Sutor, A. H.: Hämorrhagische Diathese beim Morbus Wilson. Plasmatische oder thrombocytäre Genese? Mschr. Kinderheilk. *121*:386–388, 1973.
49. Czlonkowska, A., and Konopka, L.: Cr-51 labeled erythrocyte survival time in Wilson's disease. Pol. Tyg. Lek. *42*:1638–1640, 1972.
50. Rosenfield, N., Grand, R. J., Watkins, J. B., Ballantine, T. V. N., and Levey, R. H.: Cholelithiasis and Wilson's disease. J. Pediatr. *92*:210–213, 1978.
51. Weinstein, M. P., Iannini, P. B., Stratton, C. W., and Eickhoff, T. C.: Spontaneous bacterial peritonitis. Amer. J. Med. *64*:592, 1978.
52. Starzl, T. Personal communication.
53. Lygren, T.: Hepatolenticular degeneration (Wilson's disease) and juvenile cirrhosis in the same family. Lancet *1*:275–276, 1959.
54. Vachon, A., Paliard, P., Barthe, J., Grimaud, J. A., Peyrol, G. L., and Reiss, Th.: Les étapes des l'atteinte hépatique de la dégénérescence hépatolenticulaire: lésions précoces, hypertension portale et dégénérescence cancereuse. A propos de 4 observations. Lyon Méd. *230*:591–598, 1973.
55. Kamakura, K., Kimura, S., Igarashi, S., Fujiwara, K., Oda, T., Yoshitoshi, Y., and Shoti, S.: A case of Wilson's disease with hepatoma. J. Jap. Soc. Int. Med. *64*:232–238, 1975.
56. Terao, H., Itakura, H., Nakata, K., Kono, K., Muro, T., Furukawa, R., Kusumoto, M., Munehisa, T., Nagataki, S., Ishii, N., Koji, T., and Hirama, M.: An autopsy case of hepatocellular carcinoma in Wilson's disease. Acta Hepatol. Jap. *23*:439–445, 1982.
57. Sakai, K., Murata, N., Katsuyoshi, C., and Yasuhiro, Y.: Effect of copper administration on the incorporation of ^{3}H-thymidine into the liver DNA of rats stimulated by dimethylnitrosamine and diethylnitrosamine. Carcinogenesis *2*:1261–1266, 1981.
58. Black, M., and Billing, B. H.: Hepatic bilirubin UDP–glucuronyl transferase activity in liver disease and Gilbert's syndrome. N. Engl. J. Med. *280*:1266–1271, 1969.

CHAPTER 8

THE CENTRAL NERVOUS SYSTEM: CLINICAL NEUROLOGY

In about 40 per cent of patients with Wilson's disease, the first clinical manifestation of the illness is neurologic. More precisely, this was true of 43 of 112 of Walshe's patients[1] and of 57 of 151 of ours. Konovalov has seen neurologic manifestations begin as early as 8 years of age and as late as 41[2]; neurologic onset occurred between the ages of 9 and 40 in 28 patients studied at the Mayo Clinic[3]; and in our experience these limits have been 6 years (patient P7) and 45 years (Patient M16). Czlonkowska has reported the case of a farmer whose Wilson's disease began with tremors at age 46.[4] Although excess copper is ubiquitous in the brain, the neurologic disturbances are almost completely limited to the motor system. Sensory abnormalities or significant muscular weakness are never seen, and reflex changes are quite uncommon. Only recurrent headaches or, rarely, grand mal or partial complex seizures appear to be exceptions to the exclusively motor nature of the disease.

MODE OF NEUROLOGIC ONSET AND COURSE

The neurologic symptoms of Wilson's disease usually first make their appearance, in one or more of the following ways, during the second or third decade of life:

a. Tremor, at rest or purposive
b. Dysarthria, as scanned, hypophonic or indistinct speech
c. Drooling
d. Diminished dexterity or mild clumsiness
e. Unsteady or ungainly gait with a tendency to lurch, stagger or stumble

f. Rigidity of the mouth, arms or legs
g. Choreiform movements or small-amplitude twitches of the fingers
h. Grand mal seizures

The neurologic onset is usually insidious, with the appearance and gradual worsening of a single symptom and development of other motor abnormalities and progressive disability. But a single symptom may predominate for months or even years before others appear. Mild or moderate disability that has been constant for some time may exacerbate abruptly and dramatically, a development ascribed by some patients to emotional conflict or stress. In a patient's initial history (and subsequently if specific treatment is not given) there may be periods of significant, spontaneous and inexplicable amelioration of disease. Without decoppering treatment, however, sooner or later relapse and progression to total incapacity and death are inevitable.

Examples of these eight modes of neurologic onset of Wilson's disease, keyed to the list above, follow.

a. K2 a 23-year-old right-handed dental technician, noted a tremor of his left hand that involved his right within 6 months.

a. L3, a 23-year-old man, was embarrassed to drink coffee in a restaurant because of his tremors, which alcohol diminished.

a. An aunt of a 26-year-old woman, P3, had noted shaking of her niece's head 13 years before the diagnosis of Wilson's disease was made.

a. Despite tremors and slurred speech that had been noted at age 11, a 19-year-old man, F7, was found suitable for the Marines, only to be promptly discharged because he could not salute without shaking uncontrollably.

a. N1, an 18-year-old girl whose six years of headaches and excessive salivation had been dismissed as of no consequence, was asked in a restaurant by her escort whether he made her so nervous that she trembled.

a. Tremor of the head, developing in a 22-year-old woman, A2, was attributed to her marrying outside of her ethnic culture.

b. Because the speech of a healthy 19-year-old man, C3, was indistinct, a dentist removed all of his teeth.

b. Slurred speech in a 16-year-old girl, M2, was thought to be caused by hypertrophied tonsils, which were removed.

b. A dentist, an ophthalmologist, and a gynecologist all noted the slurred speech of a 19-year-old girl, M5, who was referred, by the last, for consultation with a neurologist, who diagnosed the symptoms as psychogenic.

b. Neighbors noted slurring of speech in a 16-year-old girl, R8, before her family was aware of it.

b. An ophthalmologist, on routine examination, saw Kayser-Fleischer rings in a 38-year-old woman, K3, who had suffered from 15 years of severe migrainous headaches and who, along with her husband and adopted children, was totally unaware of her scanned speech.

c. Drooling first appeared in a 20-year-old girl, G7; within two months, her speech became slow and monotonous.

d. R2, an 18-year-old girl who had been an excellent classical pianist, noted that her left hand was no longer able to accompany the right.

f. At age 12, M6, a boy who had had hepatitis at age 10, complained of stiffness across his shoulders; within 4 months, he could barely write or talk, and he exhibited flexion contractures of his right elbow and wrist.

g. An 18-year-old woman, R7, suffering from progressive athetosis of her entire body, had had severe migraine-like headaches at least once a week from the age of six.

a,d. A 20-year-old radio technician, P11, found he had to hold a screwdriver with both hands in order to steady it.

a,b. M14, a 32-year-old woman, had been moderately incapacitated for five years with progressive tremors, ataxia and dysarthria before she was recognized to have Wilson's disease.

d,e. Unsteady gait and impaired coordination in using tools or playing softball were the first symptoms noted by W4, a 23-year-old farmer.

b,c,f. Within months after a bout of jaundice at age 19, a "wild expression," flexion contractures of the hands, drooling, open-mouthedness, dysphagia and mutism developed in a woman, T6.

b,c,f,h. A girl, P7, who suffered from grand mal seizures beginning at age six, exhibited the rapid onset of drooling, slurred speech, open-mouthedness and rigidity in her eleventh year.

d,e,f. The handwriting of a 15-year-old girl, W1, which had been notably beautiful, deteriorated suddenly. Soon thereafter an awkward stance, a jaw that hung open, and difficulty in swallowing liquids developed.

Almost from the time of Wilson's original publication[5] it has been recognized that there are two clearly different clinical courses of the neurologic manifestations of Wilson's disease. One, in which tremors constitute the major problem, has been termed pseudosclerotic. The other, characterized by the rigidity and contractures so evident in Wilson's first patients, is generally referred to as the dystonic, or classic, form.[6, 7] Although we know of no pathogenetic basis for this difference, it is so striking that each should be described separately. In reality almost every patient with neurologic signs and symptoms suffers from tremulousness *and* dystonia, although one or the other usually predominates.

Abnormal involuntary movements afflict almost all patients with neurologic disturbances. Tremors, the commonest such movements, are of the resting, intention and postural variety (the last being most often seen), resembling a combination of parkinsonism and multiple sclerosis.

Resting tremors may be transiently attenuated by a tactile stimulus or by initiation of a voluntary movement of the affected part, and like those of parkinsonism in that they usually disappear at complete repose. They are regular, rhythmic and, particularly in fingers and wrists, slow and alternating. They can also affect proximal joints and are intensified on motion of almost any part of the body and by strong pleasant or unpleasant emotion, often spreading over the entire body in such circumstances. Wild wing-beating of the arms, occasionally seen, may be so forceful that injury is caused to the chest or abdomen.

Intention tremors are seen when a patient so affected tries to eat, dress, write, make his toilet or ambulate. They may also manifest themselves as scanned speech, titubation, dropping of objects, or clumsiness. Boudin and Pépin[8] have characterized the clinical picture of these manifestations as a "tremulousness of action": tremors, almost absent in repose, develop minimally when the patient stands and escalate into a "volitional dyskinesia" with a wide variety of involuntary movements, tremors and dystonic phenomena on intentional effort.

Postural and action tremors are more frequent than the resting variety. Postural tremors may affect the head (titubation), trunk, limbs, jaw or protruded tongue and may be elicited by administering a sharp perturbing blow to the outstretched, steady arm, which then may oscillate abnormally for 5 or 6 cycles. These tremors are also commonly enhanced in amplitude when the patient is anxious, agitated or being observed, as well as when he tries to use the affected limb or perform a skilled act. Other patients exhibit the tremor and accompanying dysmetria—characteristic of cerebellar dysfunction—only when performing a voluntary act or a finger-to-nose or heel-knee-shin test.

The typical severely tremulous patient walks with a wide gait, misplacing most steps from the spot sought and swinging his arms asynchronously and usually with too great an amplitude. His speech is scanned. Drinking, eating or even picking up a cup or glass may be impossible. Handwriting is generally a totally illegible scrawl with a word spread over a third or more of the page. Sleep generally brings respite from both resting and intention tremors.

Choreiform movements of the entire body are very unusual in Wilson's disease. In our patient R7, these had confined her to a bed and chair existence for a year, were athetoid in character, and were so continual that her skin was abraded by being rubbed against bed sheets. Fortunately, her movements ceased during sleep and disappeared after several months of penicillamine therapy.

In the dystonic Wilsonian patient, who may initially suffer only from muscular cramps, the extrapyramidal disorder may merely be a localized or general resistance to passive movement. Plastic or cog-wheel rigidity can sometimes be elicited by flexing and extending the elbow or wrist while the patient concentrates on alternately opening and closing his contralateral fist. When dystonia (more accurately hypertonia) is diffusely generalized, it affects the antigravity muscles, those of the neck and face, the muscles of the spinal gutters, and particularly the proximal and extensor limb muscles, the last not infrequently leading to an equinovarus foot.

Like the tremors, the dystonia of a patient is variable, again being usually absent or minimal in repose and increasing on volitional movements. Talking, for example, may be accompanied by a variety of facial grimaces, stereotyped gestures, or rhythmic movements of the hands, feet or trunk, which appear to be helping the patient articulate.

The typical dystonic patient, if he can ambulate at all, walks stiffly with head bent slightly back, mouth open, teeth protruding, and saliva ropily dripping from his mouth or onto a gauze or tissue held by hand or stuffed, gaglike, between his teeth. A fixed grin is commonly seen. Speech is generally difficult or impossible to understand, and requests for repetitions often frustrate the patient, who may angrily refuse to try to talk or may break into a long inspiratory gargling or a high-pitched cry. Interference with swallowing—caused in part by the hypertonia and spasm of mouth, throat and neck musculature—may be so severe that tube feeding is necessary. Later, the fingers may be flexed so forcibly into the palms that they cannot be even passively extended; the patient may fall stiffly on trying to sit or arise from a chair or bed; the equinovarus foot may form a continual straight line with the lower leg; and the contractures of the jaw, hands or feet may require surgical intervention. The open-mouthedness of the dystonic patient is generally associated with protrusion of the upper teeth and poor dental and gingival health. The dystonia may also be seen as masklike facies, bradykinesia or plasticity of various muscles. The "rire spasmodique" of Boudin and Pépin is the fixed, humorless smile that is commonly associated with the high-pitched, monotonous whine that is between a cry and a laugh.

NEUROLOGIC BASIS OF THE CLINICAL PICTURE

It is obvious from the foregoing that the motor disability of patients with Wilson's disease can be very profound and totally incapacitating. It is primarily, but not exclusively, the result of dysfunction of the basal ganglia and the cerebellum. It is *not* due to any significant degree of muscle weakness. Muscle atrophy or weakness, such as is caused by lesions of motor neurones of the brain stem and spinal cord, is never seen. Nor is progressive spastic paraparesis or quadriparesis (characteristic of lesions affecting upper motor neurones with predominant involvement of descending motor pathways) ever seen in Wilson's disease, and disturbance of sphincter and autonomic function (characteristic of demyelinating disorders) is extremely unusual. Weakness, if present at all, is mild and always insignificant in comparison to the disability caused by the clumsiness, loss of dexterity and motor control, and slowing of voluntary movement that are commonly so marked in patients with Wilson's disease.

The corticospinal and corticobulbar pathways, further discussed below in relation to dysarthria, are occasionally affected to some extent; muscle stretch (deep tendon) reflexes may be abnormally enhanced and spread; sustained or unsustained clonus may be elicited at the ankle; and the response to plantar stimulation may be extension. It seems unlikely that dysfunction of the corticospinal pathways causes more than minimal loss of fine motor control, since the hypertonus observed in limb and axial muscles generally has the character of rigidity ascribed to dysfunction of the extrapyramidal system, rather than spasticity, despite the common use of the latter word in clinical descriptions of Wilson's disease.

The absence of sensory disturbances in Wilson's disease is striking: olfaction, vision, taste, auditory and vestibular functions, as well as somatic sensations, are all normal, in contrast to the severe disturbance of motor functions. Most remarkably, perhaps, sensation over the face, mediated by the fifth cranial nerve, is completely unaffected in patients with disabling disturbances of the motor functions of the same nerve. Although Wilson[5] and most authors since have said that ocular motility is spared, complaints of diplopia and findings of limitation or absence of convergence; slowed, ratchety, cogwheel (or absence of) pursuit movements; ptosis; sluggish or absent pupillary reflexes; transient external ophthalmoplegia; and/or limitation of upward gaze have been present in a number of our patients and those of other authors.[9, 10, 11, 12] (see Chapter 10.) One of our patients, J3, who could elevate her gaze only a few degrees above the horizontal, regained about 30 degrees of upward gaze after a year of treatment with D-penicillamine, suggesting that the abnormality was indeed due to her Wilson's disease.

The effects of the basal gangliar disturbance on cranial nerves V, VII, IX, XI and XII produce the most distressing neurologic manifestations of Wilson's disease—the parkinsonian fixed expression; the decreased frequency of blinking; the prolonged or permanent dystonic smile; the constantly open mouth; dysarthria; dysphagia; profuse drooling; and the retraction of the upper lip, and lower jaw—all hallmarks of classic Wilson's disease.

Disturbances in speech trouble patients perhaps more than any other single neurologic abnormality. In large part this is because the dysarthria is so frequently misinterpreted as a sign of mental retardation, which is ironic, since intelligence remains virtually unaffected in the great majority of patients. A detailed analysis of the components of the dysarthria of 20 patients with Wilson's disease showed ataxic, hypokinetic and spastic elements in those whose speech was abnormal, reflecting, the authors concluded, neurologic dysfunction of the cerebellum, basal ganglia and upper motor neurones.[13] A cinematic x-ray study of nine patients with the predominantly tremulous form of the disease revealed "steplike, jerking" movements of the diaphragm that were thought to account for the scanned cerebellar speech of these patients.[14] The scanned speech of the primarily tremulous patient is usually easily understood, but the speech of the dystonic patient is not.[15] The latter may be reduced to very low volume or a whisper, with so little movement of the lips that, as Boudin and Pépin have pointed out, the patient appears to be a ventriloquist.[8] In the open-mouthed dystonic patient, the high-pitched, drawn-out, gargling cry to which we have referred may be the only sound that can be produced. Either through disgust at having to repeat a phrase time after time before his listener understands, or because dystonic dysarthria makes intelligible speech virtually impossible, the patient may ultimately become completely mute, carrying an alphabet card with which he can often spell very rapidly and express subtle ideas. In milder dystonic affliction, speech may only be dysphonic or monotonic, the former quite likely because of impaired control and coordination of the respiratory muscles required for normal voice production.

As dysarthria worsens, patients begin to complain of difficulty in swallowing.[16] Eventually the immobility of the tongue is such that food placed in the mouth cannot be manipulated and delivered to the oropharynx. If drooling is present, because of the constantly open mouth, it now becomes more profuse.

It seems quite probable that dysfunction of extrapyramidal and corticobulbar systems is the predominant cause of these disturbances of the bulbar muscles. The severe dysarthria, dysphagia, and marked slowing of voluntary movements of the face, tongue and palate (whistling is almost always impossible in the dysarthric patients) closely resemble what is seen in patients with pseudobulbar palsy, in whom it is known that there is involvement of corticobulbar pathways. Both types of patients show a similar exaggeration of emotional expression with an abnormal-sounding laugh. Involvement of the cerebellum, and perhaps of the substantia nigra, can be assumed in those patients with scanned speech; and perhaps there is involvement of the nigrostriatal pathways in those with fairly good articulation of speech that lacks volume and modulation. Hypertonus and immobility of bulbar and facial muscles, which impair articulation may be due to damage to the putamen. The relative infrequency of an increase in the jaw jerk and in other reflexes produced by stretching of facial muscles suggests that the Wilsonian patients suffer from a preponderance of extrapyramidal dysfunction rather than spasticity of bulbar muscles.

Disturbances of the motor system may be troublesome to the patient even when they appear relatively subtle to the physician. Loss of dexterity may make dressing, eating and the other activities of daily living painfully slow and difficult. Yet neurologic examination may reveal only that touching each of the fingers with the thumb, in turn, is markedly slowed, requiring enormous effort, or that alternating movements of various joints are markedly impaired.

Very rarely, hemiparesis may occur in Wilson's disease.

It is worth emphasizing that the almost complete absence of sensory changes in Wilson's disease is of considerable differential diagnostic significance, and it is worth repeating that recurrent headache is practically the only significant exception to sensory sparing. In about 10 per cent of patients with Wilson's disease the first indication of neurologic disturbance may be either headache—often severe, persisting for years or decades, described as migrainous, and sometimes associated with nausea and vomiting—or seizures. (We have not included headache as a mode of neurologic onset, for obvious reasons.) Seizures may be grand mal or partial complex. [17–21] The latter, in one of our patients, P11, almost always begin with a "brown smell," and this olfactory sensation is occasionally followed by a brief period of impaired consciousness. Boudin and Pépin describe "tonic crises" in which tetanoid trismus and opisthotonos may occur.[8] Headache generally does not disappear with otherwise successful specific decoppering treatment; seizures usually do or, if persistent, are generally less frequent and severe.

REFERENCES

1. Walshe, J. M.: Wilson's disease (hepatolenticular degeneration). *In* Handbook of Clinical Neurology. Metabolic and Deficiency Diseases of the Nervous System. Vol. 27, Part I. Ed. by Vinken, P. J., Bruyn, G. W., and Klawans, H. L. American Elsevier, New York, 1976, pp. 379–414.
2. Konovalov, N. V.: Hepatocerebral Dystrophy. Medgiz, Moscow, 1960.
3. Dobyns, W. B., Goldstein, N. P., and Gordon, H.: Clinical spectrum of Wilson's disease. (Hepatolenticular degeneration.) Mayo Clin. Proc. *54*:35–42, 1979.
4. Czlonkowska, A., and Rodo, M.: Late onset of Wilson's disease. Arch. Neurol. *38*:729–730, 1981.
5. Wilson, S. A. K.: Progressive lenticular degeneration: a familial nervous disease associated with cirrhosis of the liver. Brain *34*:295–507, 1912.
6. Denny-Brown, D.: Hepatolenticular degeneration (Wilson's disease). N. Engl. J. Med. *270*:1149–1156, 1964.
7. Greenfield, J. G., Poynton, F. J., and Walshe, F. M. R.: On progressive lenticular degeneration. (Hepatolenticular generation.) Quart. J. Med. *17*:385–403, 1923–1924.
8. Boudin, G., and Pépin, B.: Dégénérescence Hépato-Lenticulaire. Masson, Paris, 1959.
9. Heine, L.: Ueber Augenveränderungen bei Pseudosklerose. Klin. Mobl. Augenheilk. *91*:433–437, 1933.

10. Walsh, F. B., and Hoyt, W. F.: Clinical Neuro-Ophthalmology, 3rd ed., Vol. II. Williams and Wilkins, Baltimore, 1969, p. 1042.
11. Kirkham, T. H., and Kamin, D. F.: Slow saccadic eye movements in Wilson's disease. J. Neurol. Neurosurg. Psychiatr. *37*:191–194, 1974.
12. Gadoth, N., and Liel, Y.: Transient external ophthalmoplegia in Wilson's disease. Metabol. Pediat. Ophthalmol. *4*:71–72, 1980.
13. Berry, W. R., Darley, F. L., Aronson, A. E., and Goldstein, N. P.: Dysarthria in Wilson's disease. J. Speech Hearing Res. *17*:169–183, 1974.
14. Mavlov, L., and Elenkov, P.: Role of ataxic tremor of the diaphragm in the pathogenesis of cerebellar speech disorders. Zh. Nevropatol. Psikhiatr. *71*:1787–1789, 1971.
15. Dordain, M., and Chevrie-Muller, C.: Voice and speech in Wilson's disease. Folia Phoniat. *29*:217–232, 1977.
16. Haggstrom, G., and Hirschowitz, B. I.: Disordered esophageal motility in Wilson's disease. J. Clin. Gastroenterol. *2*:273–275, 1980.
17. Smith, C. K., and Mattson, R. H.: Seizures in Wilson's disease. Neurology *17*:1121–1123, 1967.
18. Passouant, P., Mirouze, J., Mary, P., Baldy-Moulinier, M., and Mahini, P.: Epilepsie de type psycho-moteur manifestatior évolutive d'un cas maladie de Wilson. J. Méd. Montpellier *4*:147–149, 1969.
19. Capon, A., Huysman, E., Moerman, Ch., and Toth, L. Q.: Manifestations convulsives dans la maladie de Wilson. Etude életrochimique d'un cas. Arch. Neurol. Neurochir. Psych. *113*:209–225, 1973.
20. Ledić, P., Sepčić, J., Antončić, N., and Sepić, D.: Epilepsija i hepatolentikularna degeneracija. Nevropsihiatrija *23*:165–168, 1975.
21. Westmoreland, B. F., Goldstein, N. P., and Klass, D. W.: Wilson's disease. Electroencephalographic and evoked potential studies. Mayo Clin. Proc. *49*:401–404, 1974.

CHAPTER 9

THE CENTRAL NERVOUS SYSTEM: PSYCHIATRIC DISORDERS

In what was probably his last review of his disease[1] Wilson wrote, "Too much must not be made of these psychotic symptoms," referring, by "psychotic," to the totality of mental symptoms seen. He describes such disturbances as infrequent and ephemeral and writes about them, as he does about the liver, somewhat irritably, as though psychiatric or hepatic symptomatology were contaminating the neurologic purity of progressive lenticular degeneration. Yet in his original monograph of 42 years earlier he had written, "Of considerable interest are the psychical symptoms," which he had described in eight of twelve patients. Their "importance, therefore, must not be understimated."[2]

In the last 70 years, it has become clear that Wilson's initial assessment of the importance of mental symptoms was truer than his last.[3–7] Almost every patient with clinically manifest Wilson's disease suffers, at some time during the course of his disease, from organic dementia[7, 15–18]; a psychoneurosis[6, 22, 23, 26]; a manic-depressive or schizophrenic psychosis,[7, 13, 17, 19, 21, 23, 26–28] or a disorder impossible to distinguish from these[5]; bizarre behavioral abnormalities, often characterized by impulsivity[6–9, 12, 13, 15, 23, 26] and occasionally extending to criminal behavior[28a]; or a combination of any of the foregoing.[10, 11, 14, 15, 17, 20, 26]

Organic dementia may cause a general learning disability often manifest in a rather sudden deterioration in the quality of schoolwork of adolescents, an inability to concentrate or read, memory loss or confusion about life and its activities.

Anxiety, chronic or as acute attacks; conscious or subconscious fears elicited by awareness, often vague, of the catastrophe that is brewing; preoccupation with sexuality or death; moderate depression; insomnia; compulsive, obsessive or phobic behavior and thoughts; or suicidal attempts are—particularly if unaccompanied by neurologic signs—almost always interpreted as functional psychiatric disturbances.

Paranoid delusions, manic-depressive disease and severe depression represent schizophrenic or cyclothymic disorders that differ so little, if at all, from the idiopathic psychoses that Wilson's disease is virtually never suspected.

Impulsive, inappropriate or grossly antisocial behavior—exemplified by violent assault, tantrums, exhibitionism, sexual promiscuity, lying or thievery—is not uncommon. Behavioral changes may take the form of frequent, prolonged daydreaming; intense interpersonal friction, notably between adolescent patients and their parents; poor judgment, not uncommonly having to do with money matters; alcoholism, sometimes resulting from the patient's awareness that tremulousness is lessened by a drink or two; or an ill-defined, but all too obvious, personality change. Patients with this mental symptomatology are often diagnosed as psychopathic personalities, with the recommendation that they be institutionalized, as, indeed, some are.

Devastating psychiatric disease is often caused, at least in part, by the profound effects that the neurologic symptomatology produces on patients' sexual attractiveness. The open-mouthed, drooling, masklike face, usually accompanied by a characteristic foul odor to the breath, and the ill-kempt appearance and dirtiness of the entire body, stemming from the dystonia or tremulousness that makes them unable to care for or groom themselves effectively, all too frequently result in a sexually (and socially) grimly repulsive individual. The consequent frustrations of such a patient, who cannot talk, walk, eat or kiss, become overwhelming, because their intellectual capacities and emotional sensitivities are generally little, if at all, diminished. One girl of 20, P5, reduced within a year of her marriage to just such mute, total disability, commented after a remarkable therapeutic response to decoppering therapy that "the most frustrating part of this whole experience is having intelligence and not being able to communicate—except by spelling on an alphabet card—because people prejudge you as an idiot."

Similar total disability and consequent physical unattractiveness apparently convinced an adolescent girl, M5, that she would be unable to date boys. She proclaimed to her parents that she was a lesbian and began a relationship with a girl, terminating it when therapy had restored her to a chic, charming and attractive person.

In perhaps 10 to 25 per cent of all patients with Wilson's disease, one or another of these disturbances may be its first clinical manifestation.[10, 11, 14, 17, 24, 26] Particularly true of dementia, as Hall first pointed out,[18] but occasionally of the psychiatric disturbances as well, it is often difficult to know whether the mental illness is real or whether the dysarthria, drooling, dystonia, open-mouthedness and inappropriate laughing and crying have deceived the physician into interpreting neurologic dysfunction as mental illness. Conversely, in 40 to 50 per cent of patients the initial and presenting neurologic manifestations may be so severe that accompanying psychiatric disturbances may be overlooked. Neurologic improvement, induced by decoppering therapy, may uncover distressing mental symptoms in these patients.

We believe that the emotional and mental disturbances seen in Wilson's disease are the results of both the direct toxic effects of the widespread cerebral deposits of copper on higher integrative brain centers and patients' reactions to the somatic (particularly the neurologic) effects of copper toxicosis. It is presently impossible to determine the relative importance of either factor in an individual patient.[5]

The same uncertainty exists in Parkinson's[29] and Huntington's disease,[30, 31] each of which, like Wilson's disease, is an organic brain disorder with a characteristic neurologic symptomatology, an organic mental syndrome (dementia) and/or a range of neuropsychiatric disturbances generally indistinguishable from classic functional neuroses, depressive disorders or schizophrenia.

Although excess copper is present in all parts of the brain (see Table 4–1), the selective character of the psychiatric manifestations of Wilson's disease, like that of the neurologic, indicates that some sites of central nervous system functions are more susceptible to copper toxicity than others. Behavioral disturbances, for example, are extremely common and are of the kinds associated with frontal lobe disturbances. Yet agnostic, apraxic, and aphasic phenomena are rather unusual in Wilson's disease, although there appear to be no significant differences in the concentrations of copper in the parietal, temporal and occipital lobes (where these functions are believed to be regulated) from that in the frontal lobe. Hallucinations and delusions, although not uncommon in generalized organic brain disturbances, are very unusual in Wilson's disease. The spontaneous laughing and crying, often with prolonged inspiratory whooping sounds, that Wilson described have become almost a hallmark of the disease but are seen in less than half of the patients.[2]

Clinical examination or biochemical measurements can unequivocally confirm or rule out the diagnosis of Wilson's disease once it is thought of, but only when it *is* thought of.[14] Unfortunately, both in patients whose first clinical manifestations are psychiatric and in those with initial neurologic disturbances who are referred to a psychiatrist by a physician who can find no organic cause for their symptoms and signs, Wilson's disease is not suspected often enough by psychiatrists. In both types of patients the eventual appearance or progression of the neurologic symptomatology generally leads to uneasiness on the part of the psychiatrist, who thereupon undertakes investigations to uncover some organic brain or somatic disease. But these investigations will prove fruitless unless suspicion of Wilson's disease leads, at least, to a determination of the serum concentration of ceruloplasmin and a slit-lamp examination of the eyes for Kayser-Fleischer rings.

Brief summaries of nine of our patients follow.

An 18-year-old girl, M5, was referred to a psychiatrist for treatment of vague complaints for which extensive metabolic investigation could reveal no cause. Progressive neurologic disability was persistently interpreted solely in psychodynamic terms for three years despite her referral to a neurologist by her gynecologist, who suspected multiple sclerosis because of slurred speech (also noted by her dentist and ophthalmologist). Only three months later, by which time she had become virtually unable to walk, talk, or feed herself, was the diagnosis of Wilson's disease suspected and confirmed, as she later described: "It began with severe leg cramps in tenth grade. I remember crying . . . being fitted for fancy arch supports . . . couldn't seem to

get enough sleep, but there were family problems and I chalked it up to that. I stopped menstruating. My body was going on strike. Out of high school four months, I lay in a hospital bed. Barium enema, GI series, brain scan, liver scan, x-rays, glucose tolerance test, renal testing, three weeks of testing. According to the tests, I was fine. It was obvious by looking at me something was wrong. I began psychotherapy. For a year I improved. Then my speech began to slur and I nose-dived. My hands shook. My sense of balance came and went. I became a depressed lethargic slob. I forgot how to tie my shoe, hold a pen, swallow, walk. I admitted myself to the hospital under my psychiatrist's care. Tests, consultations, interviews, conferences. The staff was baffled. I was sicker each day. Panic, worry, helplessness. No one knew what to do. We were all skidding towards my death. I was in a fog. Doctors, ambulance, New York doctor, New York hospital. I have Wilson's disease. I have who?"

Treatment with penicillamine and BAL was astonishingly successful in ameliorating her neurologic disability. Within a year of its institution she was able to maintain her own apartment, drive a car and enroll in college. But recurrent depression, focused on the two years she felt had been lost from her life, led her to request hospitalization to prevent suicide, which she accomplished in the hospital 16 months after the diagnosis of Wilson's disease had been made.

From the age of 24 this man, L3, suffered from persistent compulsive voyeurism that began after he glimpsed the naked wife of a fellow air force officer. Following arrest, jail, and a suicide attempt, psychotherapy was initiated. Tremors and then incoordination, first noted at age 27, progressed. But psychotherapy continued, and not until he was 30 did an internist suspect Wilson's disease. Decoppering therapy with BAL and penicillamine—with continued but less frequent psychotherapy—was followed by complete remission of all neurologic and psychiatric signs and symptoms. Taking penicillamine alone for the last 20 years, he is married, the father of three children, and the president of a prosperous business.

When she was 26 this woman, C2, underwent the first of several hospitalizations for classic manic episodes. Three years later, following a miscarriage, tremors developed and led to the diagnosis of Wilson's disease. With the institution of penicillamine therapy, which she has taken every day for the last 17 years, her tremors have completely disappeared and her manic episodes, though recurring every two or three years, are less frequent and severe than before treatment of her Wilson's disease.

At 25 this woman, T4, began to suffer from fainting, shakiness and depression, which were diagnosed as nervous fatigue. An impulsive slashing of her wrists and psychotic delusions were followed by inpatient and outpatient psychiatric treatment until the development of severe neurologic disability two years later, when the diagnosis of Wilson's disease was made. Seven years of penicillamine therapy have left her with only minimal dysarthria, incoordination and dystonia. She is married and holds a responsible career job in government.[14]

This man, S6, was well until, at age 27, cyclic depressions and manic periods alternated. After one year of inpatient and outpatient psychiatric care, domestic strife and separation from his wife, he was admitted to a diagnostic clinic, where, with minimal neurologic

findings, the diagnosis of Wilson's disease was suspected and confirmed. Two years of penicillamine treatment, accompanied by psychotherapy and psychotropic medications (the last causing transient, mild tardive dyskinesia that complicated evaluation of his Wilsonian neurologic disease), have resulted in disappearance of his mild neurologic manifestations but, unfortunately, further progression of his psychiatric disturbances.

At 18 this boy, L4, was hospitalized in a psychiatric institution for hostility, impulsivity and grandiose ideas. He asked his parents to bring him his clarinet so that, like a Pied Piper, he could lead all the patients off the ward. Despite the appearance of slurred speech, micrographia and tremors, noted by a number of physicians at age 20, and the presence of Kayser-Fleischer rings in his blue eyes, psychotherapy alone was continued for another three years, by which time his neurologic Wilson's disease was irreversible. Vigorous decoppering therapy had no appreciable beneficial effect, and his disease progressed to total incapacity, anarthria and death.

Unexplained hepatosplenomegaly was noted when this girl, F3, was 9. Tremors, appearing at 15, were diagnosed as psychogenic, and she began psychoanalytic treatment. At 17, an internist, to whom she was taken because her mother suspected organic disease, saw her Kayser-Fleischer rings. Continual penicillamine therapy for the last 25 years has resulted in neurologic normality but has left her suffering from constant anxiety, phobias, and compulsions punctuated by two psychotic episodes requiring hospitalization.

When she was 18 this woman, R2, who had been able to play Beethoven piano sonatas at 12, noted that her left hand was unable to follow her right. Soon her academic work deteriorated and she was admitted to several diagnostic clinics—medical and psychiatric—at all of which she was told she was suffering from neurotic or psychotic illness. She refused the suggestion at her last admission that she enter a state mental hospital and continued outpatient psychotherapy until, when tremors, drooling and open-mouthedness had become incapacitating, a physician in a clinic suspected the cause of her condition. Intensive decoppering treatment has completely eliminated all of her neurologic manifestations, although persistent psychoneurosis and her immature ego have led her into an unworkable marriage; prevented her, despite rather high intelligence, from any gainful work; and kept her from enjoying her genuine musical talent.

At 22, shortly after her marriage, this woman, S7, complained of persistent dysphagia that was attributed to a globus hystericus induced by her having been compelled to practice fellatio. Because psychotherapy resulted in no improvement in her dysphagia, she was hospitalized with a diagnosis of schizophrenia and given electroconvulsive treatments. By the time Wilson's disease was diagnosed she had become totally incapacitated, and has remained so—apparently decerebrate—despite intensive decoppering therapy that has been continued for more than eight years.

The foregoing has practical importance for patients and their psychotherapists for four reasons:

1. Wilson's disease may present with striking behavioral and psychiatric manifestations *before* the appearance of any movement disorder.

2. A movement disorder due to undiagnosed Wilson's disease may be erroneously—and tragically—discounted as being part of a nonspecific psychiatric disturbance or as having been caused by pharmacologic treatment of such a disturbance.

3. If the diagnosis is not made sufficiently early, none of the clinical manifestations of Wilson's disease, including the psychiatric, may be reversible by decoppering or other therapies.

4. Psychiatric disorders arising from Wilson's disease can be successfully treated only if specific therapy is directed at the underlying disturbance in copper metabolism. Psychotherapy, and the milder tranquilizing or antidepressant drugs are generally essential adjuvants to treatment with penicillamine when psychiatric disturbances are more than minimal. But we and others believe that electroconvulsive treatment and insulin coma are *never*—and drugs such as haloperidol, lithium salts, and propranolol are rarely—of value in Wilson's disease.[32, 33]

Obviously the overwhelming majority of psychiatrically ill patients do not suffer from Wilson's disease. A patient's psychotherapist should, however, determine the concentration of ceruloplasmin in serum and the presence or absence of Kayser-Fleischer rings to rule out the possibility of Wilson's disease—particularly in a patient under age 40—if there is a family history of the disorder, if the patient has a history of unexplained liver disease, if the patient is not responding satisfactorily to psychiatric treatment or if neurologic signs and symptoms supervene.

REFERENCES

1. Wilson, S. A. K.: Progressive lenticular degeneration. *In* Neurology. Ed. by Bruce, A. N. Williams and Wilkins, Baltimore, 1955, pp. 941–967.
2. Wilson, S. A. K.: Progressive lenticular degeneration: A familial nervous disease associated with cirrhosis of the liver. Brain, *34*:295–507, 1912.
3. Scheinberg, I. H. Psychosis associated with hereditary disorders. *In* American Handbook of Psychiatry, 2nd ed., vol. 4. Ed. by Reiser, M. R. Organic Disorders and Psychosomatic Medicine, Chapter 16, Basic Books, New York, 1968, pp. 404–411.
4. Scheinberg, I. H. A psychogenetic anecdote. Psychosom. Med. *37*:368–371, 1975.
5. Beard, A. W.: The association of hepatolenticular degeneration with schizophrenia. Acta Psych. Neurol. Scand. *34*:411–426, 1959.
6. Goldstein, N. P., Ewert, M. A., Randall, R. V., and Gross, J. B.: Psychiatric aspects of Wilson's disease (hepatolenticular degeneration): Results of psychometric tests during long-term therapy. Amer. J. Psychiat. *124*:1155–1561, 1968.
7. Konovalov, N. V.: Hepatocerebral Dystrophy. Medgiz, Moscow, 1960.
8. Steinmann, I.: Genealogische Ermittlungen in 4 Familien mit Westphal-Wilsonscher Pseudosklerose; neurologische und psychische Besonderheiten im klinischen Bild bei 4 erkrankten Geschwisterpaaren. Arch. Psych. *105*:514–538, 1936.
9. Schwyn, H.: Über zwei Fälle von Wilsoncher Krankheit bei einem Geschwisterpaar. Schweiz. Arch. Neurol. Psychiat. *40*:221–241, 1937.
10. Findlay, D.: La maladie de Wilson. Histoire d'un cas. Can. Psychiatr. Assoc. J., *21*:117–121, 1976.
11. Basquin, M.: Hystérie, schizophrénie, maladie de Wilson. Rev. Neuropsychiat infant. *23*:195–200, 1975.
12. Koch, G.: Kasuistischer Beitrag für Erblichkeit der Westphal-Wilsonschen Pseudosklerose. Arch. Psychiat. *112*:101–109, 1940.
13. Kunath, B.: Zur Psychopathologie der hepato-zerebralen Degeneration. Fortschr. Neurol. Psychiat. *2*:91–106, 1969.
14. Cartwright, G.: Diagnosis of treatable Wilson's disease. N. Engl. J. Med. *298*:1347–1350, 1978.
15. Hayek, H. W., Knoll, E., and Widhalm, S.: Über das organische Psychosyndrom bei Morbus Wilson. Mschr. Kinderheilk. *121*:679–683, 1973.
16. Poch, G. F., and Martin, A. J.: Un caso de degeneracion hepatolenticular con manifestaciones predominantemente psiquicas. Pren. Med. Argent. *53*:1119–1121, 1966.

17. Grigorieva, N. K. Psychiatric manifestations in children with hepatolenticular degeneration. Zh. Nevropatol. (Moscow) *72*:1568–1570, 1972.
18. Hall, H. C.: La Dégénérescence Hépato-Lenticulaire Maladie de Wilson—Pseudo-Sclérose. Masson, Paris, 1921.
19. Lisak, A.: Ein Fall von Wilson-Pseudosklerose mit katatonem Symptomenkomplex. Schweiz. Med. Wschr. *19*:161–163, 1938.
20. Schmidt, M.: Etudes sur la pathogenèse de la dégénérescence hépato-lenticulaire. Acta Psychiat. Neurol. Kbh. *5*:163–165, 1930.
21. Gysin, W. M., and Cooke, E. T.: Unusual mental symptoms in a case of hepatolenticular degeneration. Dis. Nerv. Sys. *11*:3–7, 1950.
22. Ruzickova, R., and Hauftova, D.: Psychicke poruchy u Wilsonovy choroby a jejich ovlivneni penicillaminovou terapii. Čs. Psychiat. *63*:236–242, 1967.
23. Singer, L., Sichel, J.-P., Tyano, S., and Kammerer, T.: Etude des troubles psychiatriques dans un cas familial de maladie de Wilson. Anal. Medico-psychol. *1*:276–282, 1967.
24. Galvao-Bueno, A. F., Canelas, H. M., and De Jorge, F. B.: Dengeneraçao hepatolenticular: aspectos psiquiatricos, neurologicos e bioquimicos de sete casos. Rev. Paulista Med. *68*:185–202, 1966.
25. Giagheddu, M.: Le alterazioni psichiche nella degenerazione epatolenticolare. Neopsichiatria *30*:118–156, 1964.
26. Scheinberg, I. H., Sternlieb, I., and Richman, J.: Psychiatric manifestations in patients with Wilson's disease. *In* Wilson's Disease. Birth Defects, Original Article Series, Vol. IV. Ed. by Bergsma, D., Scheinberg, I. H., and Sternlieb, I. The National Foundation—March of Dimes, New York, 1968, pp. 85–87.
27. Wallauer, P., and Harbauer, H.: Zum Verlauf und zur Therapie eines jugendlichen Morbus Wilson, Dtsch. Med. Wschr. *26*:1187–1191, 1967.
28. Parada, R.: Aspectos psicopatologicos de la degeneracion hepatolenticular o enfermedad de Wilson. Rev. Chil. Neuro-Psiq. *7*:37–42, 1968.
28a. Grünberger, J., Sluga, W., and Tschabitscher, H.: Kriminelle Verhaltensstörung bei Morbus Wilson. Wien. Zschr. Nervenheilk. *24*:313–325, 1968.
29. Lieberman, A., Dziatolowski, M., Kupersmith, M., Serby, M., Goodgold, A., Korein, J., and Goldstein, M.: Dementia in Parkinson disease. Ann. Neurol. *6*:355–359, 1979.
30. Whittier, J. R.: Mental disorders with Huntington's chore. *In* American Handbook of Psychiatry, 2nd ed., Vol. 4. Ed. by Reiser, M. R. Basic Books, New York, 1975, pp. 412–417.
31. Mann, J. J., Stanley, M., Gershon, S., and Rossor, M.: Mental symptoms in Huntington's disease and a possible primary aminergic neuron lesion. Science *210*:1369–1371, 1980.
32. Tu, J-B.: The inadvisability of neuroleptic medication in Wilson's disease. Biol. Psychiat. *16*:963–968, 1981.
33. Yudofsky, S., Williams, D., and Gorman, J.: Propranolol in the treatment of rage and violent behavior in patients with chronic brain syndromes. Amer. J. Psychiat. *138*:218–220, 1981.

CHAPTER 10

THE EYE

Despite the fact that vision is never significantly affected in Wilson's disease, the diagnostic importance of excessive ocular deposits of copper, particularly in the cornea, makes the eye, after the liver and brain, the most clinically significant target organ of this disorder (Table 10–1).

EFFECTS ON THE CORNEA: THE KAYSER-FLEISCHER RING

From observations of patients with the very earliest manifestations of extrahepatic Wilson's disease—patients usually detected because a sibling has been so diagnosed—we know that Kayser-Fleischer rings first appear as a crescent in the superior corneal quadrant, followed by an inferior crescent and ultimately by completely circumferential, opaque, golden or greenish-brown rings. Always extending centrally from the limbus (rarely as much as half the corneal radius), the rings fade gradually toward the center.[5–11] In one of our patients, L7, two concentric rings were seen, with the outer one reaching the limbus. In blue- or green-eyed individuals the color and extent of the rings can generally be seen in room light or with an ordinary flashlight directed at the cornea from the side (see Color Plate 1, Figure 1). However, examination with a slit-lamp is required to see very early rings or crescents; to be certain of their presence or absence by determining if there is pigment localized in Descemet's membrane; or to characterize their appearance, which may be homogeneous, finely granular, "hammered-metal" or "oil-on-water" (see Color Plate 1, Figure 2; and Color Plate 2, Figure 3). Kayser-Fleischer rings are also seen in patients with a copper-containing intraocular foreign body,[12] or, unusually, as discussed below, in other types of liver disease.

In some patients with marked hypercupremia associated with a form of multiple myeloma there is an iridescent golden-green film in Descemet's membrane that is densest at the center of the cornea and fades to a clear area as the limbus is approached.[13–15] This distribution of what is almost

TABLE 10–1. Copper Content of Various Eye Tissues in Normal Subjects and Patients with Wilson's Disease

TISSUE	NORMAL *mcg/gdw**	*n*	WILSON'S DISEASE *mcg/gdw*	*n*	REF.
Cornea	51.6	4	281.5	2	1,2
Lens	32.3	4	49.6	2	1,2
Conjunctiva	60.9	4	619.8	2	1,2
Sclera	39.0	3	13.3	2	1,2
Uvea	65.8	3	367.9	2	1,2
Vitreous	28.6	3	277.1	2	1,2
Muscle	50.9	2	147.5	2	1,2
Optic nerve	61.1	3	235.2	2	1,2
Retina	25.8	1	258.7	1	1,2
	mcg/ml		*mcg/ml*		
Aqueous	n.v.	—	9.5	1	2
Aqueous	0.1	20	0.9–7.6	5	3
Cornea	1.2	2	1.2–73.1	7	4
Cornea					
Superior limbus	2.7	1	176	3	4a
Inferior limbus	3.5	1	150	3	4a
Medial limbus	3.4	1	156	3	4a
Lateral limbus	3.2	1	175	3	4a
Central area	2.6	1	185	3	4a

*mcg/gram dry weight; single values are means of eyes of n subjects.

certainly copper-containing pigment is precisely the reverse of that of Kayser-Fleischer rings. A copper-binding immunoglobulin has been isolated from one of these patients.[15]

Intermittently studied since 1908, Kayser-Fleischer rings have been considered by various investigators to be composed of silver, antimony, iron or an organic pigment of hematogenous origin.[16] The first suggestion that they might represent deposits of copper was made in 1922, and the first unambiguous demonstration of copper in a ring was made by Gerlach and Rohrschneider in 1934.[17] In 1943 Eckardt et al. found, by spectroscopy, that the corneas from two patients with Wilson's disease contained copper, zinc, and iron, none of which was detected in the normal cornea.[18] That the rings do indeed contain copper (and no significant amounts of iron or zinc) is now fully confirmed by a number of chemical, spectroscopic, histochemical, and x-ray spectroscopic analyses.[2, 4, 7, 19, 20] (Rings with the characteristic localization and appearance of Kayser-Fleischer rings but presumably caused by deposits of silver—the source of which, however, could not be identified—have been described in one patient in whom there was no evidence for an intraocular foreign body and who certainly did not have Wilson's disease.[21]) By light and electron microscopy the copper-containing granules are seen to be in as many as three discrete layers.[22] In each, round clusters of electron-dense particles are localized at anywhere between 0.6 and 2 mμ anterior to the endothelial layer of the cornea.[23, 24]

Johnson and Campbell's data[4a] suggest that the Kayser-Fleischer ring represents a complex of copper with a sulfur-containing molecule, since the central area of the cornea of patients with Wilson's disease contains as much copper as the limbus but does not contain sulfur (Table 10–1), whereas sulfur is present in Descemet's membrane.

Kayser-Fleischer rings are present in *all* patients with neurologic manifestations of Wilson's disease and in most patients with hepatic manifestations, as exemplified by six out of seven patients with rings whose Wilson's disease was first manifested as chronic active hepatitis.[25] In four asymptomatic subjects (of the 155 patients discussed in Chapter 14), discovery of the rings was the first indication that they suffered from Wilson's disease.

In 1965 we stated that the confirmed presence of a Kayser-Fleischer ring was "a sufficient criterion for the diagnosis of Wilson's disease."[26] It has since been established that this is not the case. Rings indistinguishable by slit-lamp examination from Kayser-Fleischer rings have been reported to occur in primary biliary cirrhosis,[27, 28] chronic intrahepatic[29] and extrahepatic cholestasis,[30] chronic active hepatitis[27, 31] and cryptogenic cirrhosis.[31, 32]

Golden, copper-containing rings in Descemet's membrane, indistinguishable from Kayser-Fleischer rings, can also result from copper penetrating, or applied to, the eye; these have been reported in 9 of 10 patients known to have had ocular chalcosis (the presence of an intraocular copper-containing foreign body) for periods ranging from 4 months to 29 years.[12] They have also appeared in patients with trachoma or other eye diseases for which topical copper solutions were applied as treatment.[33]

In addition to the corneal deposits occurring in some instances of multiple myeloma, an arcus senilis or juvenilis and corneal discoloration must be distinguished from Kayser-Fleischer rings. An arcus is located in the corneal stroma, not in Descemet's membrane, and always displays a clear area between its outer circumference and the limbus. Yet an erroneous diagnosis of Wilson's disease was based on rings that proved to be golden-yellow arci seniles as a result of carotenemia.[34] Nor should corneal pigmentation by bilirubin, occasionally seen in patients with long-standing jaundice,[35] be confused with Kayser-Fleischer rings, since the bilirubin is also present in the corneal stroma and does not produce the reflection from Descemet's membrane seen with genuine rings.

No matter what the pathogenesis of a Kayser-Fleischer ring is, treatment with penicillamine generally results either in its disappearance or in diminution of its size and intensity.[36, 37] Occasionally rings persist despite adequate treatment with this drug.[38] In a unique instance, fading and ultimately complete disappearance of Kayser-Fleischer rings occurred in a 14-year-old boy with Wilson's disease who underwent successful liver transplantation because of his intolerance to both penicillamine and triethylene tetramine.[36]

The fading of rings that is induced by penicillamine therapy occurs in the reverse order in which the rings appear, often completely disappearing from the medial and lateral quadrants before any noticeable diminution in their intensity occurs superiorly or inferiorly, where crescents may persist for years.[11, 39]

SUNFLOWER CATARACT

A sunflower cataract can often be seen with the ophthalmoscope as a disc-shaped opacity "about the size of the pupillary aperture, with spokes radiating toward the lens periphery like the petals of a flower."[10]It is golden, greenish, or gray (see Color Plate 2, Figure 4). With the slit-lamp, powdery deposits similar to those seen in Descemet's membrane are visible.[10, 40, 41] In Wilson's disease these cataracts form much less frequently than the Kayser-Fleischer ring. In contrast, when the ring is caused by an intraocular copper-containing foreign body it is almost always accompanied by a sunflower cataract; the latter can even be present without a Kayser-Fleischer ring.[12] A similar appearance can occur in patients with the form of multiple myeloma that causes the corneal films described above.[13, 14]

Sunflower cataracts rarely affect vision and, whether associated with Wilson's disease or chalcosis, generally diminish in intensity or disappear with penicillamine treatment.[37, 41] Structural and ultrastructural studies demonstrate that they are associated with deposits of copper in both the anterior and posterior lens capsule.[19, 42]

RETINAL CHANGES

Pillat[43] and Ling (quoted in reference 16) observed small, white retinal spots that radiated from the optic disc or macular areas in at least four patients with Wilson's disease. Since these patients were all seen before the introduction of decoppering therapy for Wilson's disease, the spots were either a coincidental finding or another manifestation of copper toxicity. In 1978 Dingle and Havener described a patient with Wilson's disease whose initial ophthalmoscopic examination was normal, but in whom very similar retinal spots developed after ten years of daily administration of one gram of penicillamine.[44] By then the lateral and medial portions of the patient's Kayser-Fleischer rings had disappeared and she was apparently well clinically, so the authors speculated that copper deficiency or a toxic effect of penicillamine might have caused the drusen-like lesions. Their inclusion of the possibility of a direct toxic effect of copper on retinal pigment epithelial cells is difficult to reconcile with the amount of penicillamine given. Segal and co-workers reported a patient with Wilson's disease and impaired dark-adaptation who exhibited discrete degenerative changes in the periphery of both retinas.[45]

EFFECTS ON CRANIAL NERVES III, IV AND VI

Goldberg and von Noorden studied ocular motility in eight patients with Wilson's disease and found only minimal and clinically insignificant staircase pursuit movements in one patient[46] (but see Chapter 8). They concluded that the normality of oculomotor movements found in all but a very few patients reflected the fact that the internal corticotectal and corticotegmental tracts that mediate descending impulses "probably avoid intimate anatomic connection with the basal ganglia and thus may not be subject to pathologic extrapyramidal influences." Klingele, Newman and Burde[47] reported a patient with Wilson's disease who suffered, at age 22, from blurred vision due to an accommodation defect that the authors believed was supranuclear in origin, agreeing with the conclusions of Goldberg and von Noorden.

REFERENCES

1. de Azevedo, M. L., and De Jorge, F. B.: Some mineral constituents of normal eye tissues (Na-K-Mg-Ca-P-Cu). Ophthalmologica *149*:43–52, 1965.
2. de Azevedo, M. L., De Jorge, F. B., and Canelas, H. M.: Moléstia de Wilson: Dosagem de minerals nos tecidos oculares. Rev. Brasil. Oftalmol. *25*:17–27, 1966.
3. Gerhard, J. P.: La cuivre de la chambre antérieure dans la maladie de Wilson. Rev. d'Oto-Neuro-Ophthalmol. *42*:316–319, 1970.
4. Belkin, M., Zeimer, R., Chazek, T., Freidman, G., and Melamed, E.: Corneal copper quantitation in Wilson's disease. Metabol. Ophthalmol. *2*:389, 1978.

4a. Johnson, R. E., and Campbell, R. J.: Wilson's disease. Electron microscopic, X-ray energy spectroscopic, and atomic absorption spectroscopic studies of corneal copper deposition and distribution. Lab. Invest. *46*:546–569, 1982.

5. Kayser, B.: Ueber einen Fall von angeborener grünlicher Verfärbung der Cornea. Klin. Monatsbl. Augenheilkd. *40*:22–25, 1902.
6. Fleischer, B.: Die periphere braun-grünliche Hornhautverfärbung als Symptom einer eigenartigen Allgemeinerkrankung. Münch. Med. Wochenschr. *56*:1120–1123, 1909.
7. Sternlieb, I.: The Kayser-Fleischer ring. Med. Radiogr. Photogr. *42*:14–15, 1966.
8. Korn, C.: L'anneau de Kayser-Fleischer. J. Génét. Hum. *15*:71–92, 1966.
9. Harry, J., and Tripathi, R.: Kayser-Fleischer ring. A pathological study. Brit. J. Ophthalmol. *54*:794–800, 1970.
10. Herron, B. E.: Wilson's disease. Ophthalmol. Sem. *1*:63–79, 1976.
11. Wiebers, D. O., Hollenhorst, R. W., and Goldstein, N. P.: The ophthalmologic manifestations of Wilson's disease. Mayo Clin. Proc. *52*:409–416, 1977.
12. Rosenthal, A. R., Marmor, M. F., and Leuenberger, P. L.: Chalcosis: A study of natural history. Ophthalmology *86*:1956–1969, 1979.
13. Lewis, R. A., Falls, H. F., and Troyer, D. O.: Ocular manifestations of hypercupremia associated with multiple myeloma. Arch. Ophthalmol. *93*:1050–1053, 1975.
14. Ellis, P. P.: Ocular deposition of copper in hypercupremia. Amer. J. Ophthalmol. *68*:423–427, 1969.
15. Baker, B. L., and Hultquist, D. E.: A copper-binding immunoglobulin from a myeloma patient. Purification, identification, and physical characterization. J. Biol. Chem. *253*:1195–1200, 1978.
16. Bothman, L., and Rolf, D. E.: The Kayser-Fleischer ring in Wilson's disease in microencephaly. Amer. J. Ophthalmol. *19*:26–33, 1936.
17. Gerlach, W., and Rohrschneider, W.: Besteht das Pigmet des Kayser-Fleischerschen Hornhautringes aus Silber? Klin. Wochenschr. *13*:48–49, 1949.
18. Eckardt, R. E., Stolzar, I. H., Adam, A. B., and Johnson, L. V.: The pigment of the Kayser-Fleischer ring. Amer. J. Ophthalmol. *26*:151–154, 1943.
19. Hanna, C., and Fraunfelder, F. T.: Lens capsule change after intraocular copper. Ann. Ophthalmol. *5*:9–22, 1973.
20. Belkin, M., Zeimer, R., Chajek, T., Friedman, G., and Melamed, E.: Non-invasive quantitation of corneal copper in hepatolenticular degeneration (Wilson's disease). Lancet *1*:391–392, 1976.
21. Whelton, M. J., and Pope, F. M.: Azure lunules in argyria. Arch. Intern. Med. *121*:267–269, 1968.
22. Liebergall, G. S.: Eye in hepatolenticular degeneration. Amer. J. Ophthalmol. *55*:1260–1263, 1963.
23. Uzman, L. L., and Jakus, M. A.: The Kayser-Fleischer ring. A histochemical and electron microscope study. Neurology *7*:341–355, 1957.
24. Johnson, B. L.: Ultrastructure of the Kayser-Fleischer ring. Amer. J. Ophthalmol. *76*:455–461, 1973.
25. Sternlieb, I., and Scheinberg, I. H.: Chronic hepatitis as a first manifestation of Wilson's disease. Ann. Intern. Med. *76*:59–64, 1972.
26. Scheinberg, I. H., and Sternlieb, I.: Wilson's disease. Ann. Rev. Med. *16*:119–134, 1965.
27. Fleming, C. R., Dickson, E. R., Wahner, H. W., Hollenhorst, R. W., and McCall, J. T.: Pigmented corneal rings in non-Wilsonian liver disease. Ann. Intern. Med. *86*:285–288, 1977.
28. Fleming, C. R., Dickson, E. R., Hollenhorst, R. W., Goldstein, N. P., McCall, J. T., and Baggenstoss, A. H.: Pigmented corneal rings in a patient with primary biliary cirrhosis. Gastroenterology *69*:220–225, 1975.
29. Kaplinsky, C., Sternlieb, I., Javitt, N., and Rotem, Y.: Familial cholestatic cirrhosis associated with Kayser-Fleischer rings. Pediatrics *65*:782–788, 1980.
30. Sternlieb, I.: Unpublished case of intrahepatic biliary calculi.
31. Frommer, D., Morris, J., Sherlock, S., Abrams, J., and Newman, S.: Kayser-Fleischer–like rings in patients without Wilson's disease. Gastroenterology *72*:1331–1335, 1977.
32. Rimola, A., Bruguera, M., and Rodes, J.: Kayser-Fleischer-like ring in a cryptogenic cirrhosis. Arch. Intern. Med. *138*:1857–1858, 1978.
33. Rosenthal, A. R., and Appleton, B.: Histochemical localization of intraocular copper foreign bodies. Amer. J. Ophthalmol. *79*:613–625, 1975.
34. Giorgio, A. J., Cartwright, G. E., and Wintrobe, M. M.: Pseudo-Kayser-Fleischer rings. Arch. Intern. Med. *113*:817–818, 1964.
35. Weinberg, L. M., Brasitus, T. A., and Lefkowitch, J. H.: Fluctuating Kayser-Fleischer–like rings in a jaundiced patient. Arch. Intern. Med. *141*:246–247, 1981.
36. Schoenberger, M., and Ellis, P. P.: Disappearance of Kayser-Fleischer rings after liver transplantation. Arch. Ophthalmol. *97*:1914–1915, 1979.

37. Delbecque, Ph., Sourdille, J., and Delthil, S.: Traitement de al chalcose oculaire d'origine traumatique par la pénicillamine. Bull. Mém. Soc. Fr. Ophtalmol. *79*:272–282, 1966.
38. Mitchell, A. M., and Heller, G. L.: Changes in Kayser-Fleischer ring during treatment of hepatolenticular degeneration. Arch. Ophthalmol. *80*:622–625, 1968.
39. Sussman, W., and Scheinberg, I. H.: Disappearance of Kayser-Fleischer rings. Arch. Ophthalmol. *82*:738–741, 1969.
40. Rosen, E.: Copper within the eye: With the report of a case of typical sunflower cataract of the right eye and copper cataract involving the posterior capsule of the left eye. Amer. J. Ophthalmol. *32*:248–252, 1949.
41. Cairns, J. E., Williams, H. P., and Walshe, J. M.: "Sunflower cataract" in Wilson's disease. Brit. Med. J. *3*:95–96, 1969.
42. Tso, M. O. M., Fine, B. S., and Thorpe, H. E.: Kayser-Fleischer ring and associated cataract in Wilson's disease. Amer. J. Ophthalmol. *79*:479–488, 1975.
43. Pillat, A.: Changes in the eyegrounds in Wilson's disease (pseudosclerosis). Amer. J. Ophthalmol. *16*:1–6, 1933.
44. Dingle, J., and Havener, W. H.: Ophthalmoscopic changes in a patient with Wilson's disease during long-term penicillamine therapy. Ann. Ophthalmol. *10*:1227–1230, 1978.
45. Segal, P., Ruszkowski, M., Berger, S., and Masiak, M.: Abortive form of Wilson's syndrome: with dark adaptation disturbances. Amer. J. Ophthalmol. *19*:26–33, 1936.
46. Goldberg, M. F., and von Noorden, G. K.: Ophthalmologic findings in Wilson's hepatolenticular degeneration. Arch. Ophthalmol. *75*:162–170, 1966.
47. Klingele, T. G., Newman, S. A., and Burde, R. M.: Accommodation defect in Wilson's disease. Amer. J. Ophthalmol. *90*:22–24, 1980.

CHAPTER 11

THE KIDNEY

Following the almost simultaneous discoveries, in 1948, by Mandelbrote and his co-workers, of an excessive amount of urinary copper[1] and, by Uzman and Denny-Brown, of amino-aciduria[2] in patients with Wilson's disease, it soon became evident that the toxicity of copper, as an instance of heavy metal poisoning, caused not only the amino-aciduria but enough other renal tubular defects[3–14] to constitute the Fanconi syndrome.[15] No convincing evidence has been presented for the converse hypothesis, since abandoned,[16] that this renal lesion is the primary genetic defect in Wilson's disease that results in secondary defects in copper metabolism.[17]

PATHOLOGY

Except for urinary calculi or nephrocalcinosis (Fig. 11–1) there are no gross lesions of the urinary tract associated with Wilson's disease

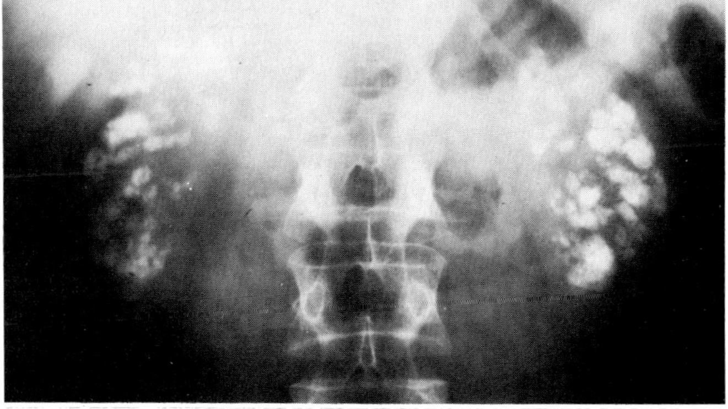

Figure 11–1. The radiopaque calcium deposits in both kidneys of patient B3, shown here at age 38 years, have increased, when compared with an examination 14 years earlier (see reference 10), without causing significant change in renal function. X-ray without contrast.

except that the kidneys of patients dying of severe hepatic insufficiency are generally enlarged and icteric.

Most of the histopathologic changes described have been in the tubules, a fact consonant with the predominance of functional tubular abnormalities. Even when such abnormalities are present, however, there may be no histologic findings, as illustrated by the absence of even a single significant change in 19 renal biopsy specimens, a number of which were obtained from patients with functional renal abnormalities.[15, 18–20] Hypercellularity of glomeruli is occasionally seen (Fig. 11–2). Renal dysfunction often complicates hepatic insufficiency, the commonest cause of death in Wilson's disease. Therefore, it is highly unlikely that any of the pathologic observations made at autopsy of these patients—when bile, granular or hyaline casts and tubular degeneration with fat deposition in, and vacuolization and sloughing of, epithelial cells may be seen[21–25]—is specific for Wilson's disease.

The possible diagnostic significance of microscopic deposits of calcium in the tubules is noteworthy, since these are the most frequent pathologic finding (Figs. 11–2 and 11–3)[26–28] and are occasionally seen in biopsy specimens. Nephrocalcinosis, generally with focal chronic pyelonephritis, has also been seen in biopsy as well as autopsy specimens (note references 10 and 29 and patients B3 and O2). Flattening of the postglomerular proximal tubule[30] and ringlike nuclei in epithelial cells[22,31] have been described in several cases.

Histologic examination of a renal biopsy sample obtained from a 19-year-old Thai man, I1, with severe neurologic Wilson's disease but no

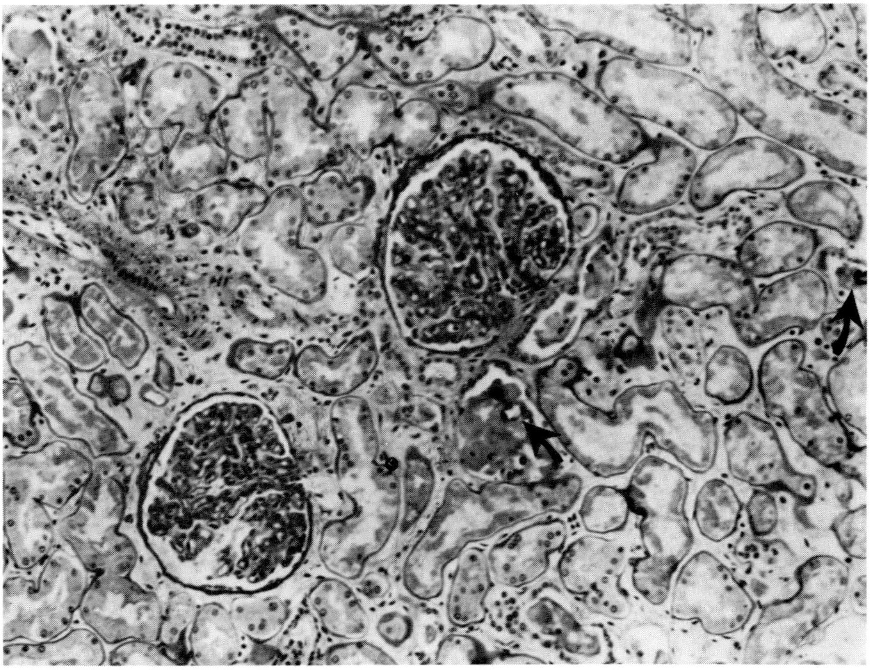

Figure 11–2. There are two hypercellular glomeruli in this field. Certain tubules contain discrete calcifications *(arrows)*. Autopsy specimen of kidney. Patient R4. PAS stain. × 140.

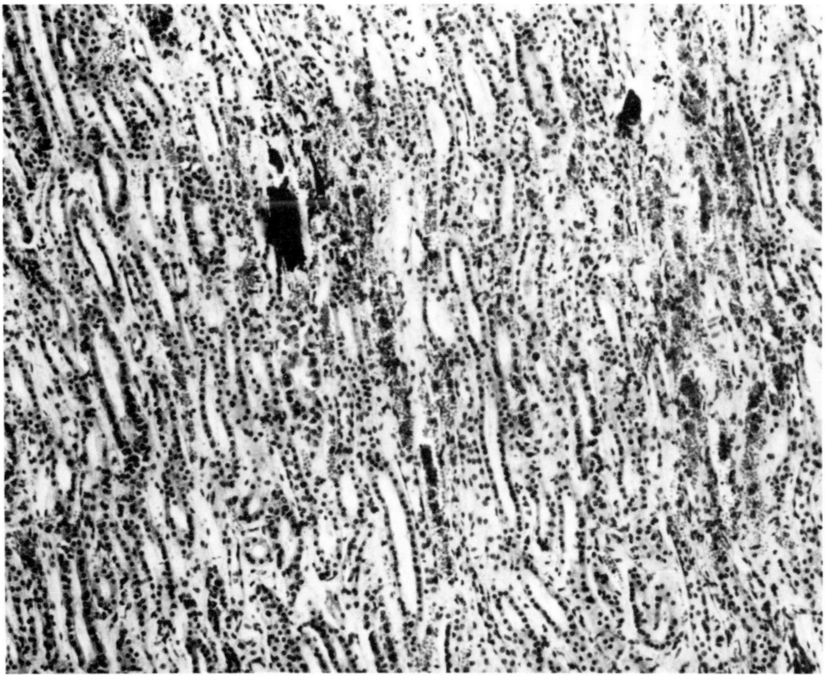

Figure 11–3. Scattered tubular calcifications in the renal medulla. Autopsy specimen of kidney. Patient S16. Hematoxylin-eosin. × 100.

history or evidence of even minimal renal or hepatic dysfunction revealed most glomeruli to be swollen and hypercellular, with focal capillary lumen obliteration in some glomerular lobules and one totally hyalinized glomerulus (Fig. 11–4). The tubules, vessels and interstitium were not remarkable. Except for thickening of the basement membrane, capsular fibrosis, and hyalinization of a few glomeruli in a biopsy sample[31a] and fibrosis of a few glomeruli in one patient at autopsy,[32] we are unaware of other reports of glomerular pathology in untreated patients.

Despite the paucity of histopathologic changes, there are several reasons for believing that the functional renal disturbances reflect toxicity of copper. First, the mean copper concentration in the kidneys, at autopsy, of eight of our untreated patients with Wilson's disease was 904 mcg/gdw (range: 100 to 2045), compared with a normal concentration of 15 (range: 5 to 36).[33]* Second, the functional renal abnormalities of a number of patients have disappeared or improved with the administration of D-penicillamine[10, 34–37] and recurred when its administration was discontinued.[38] Third, rubeanic acid staining has shown that the intracytoplasmic granules in the tubular epithelium of patients contain copper.[21, 26] It is also worth noting that cirrhosis of the liver, a sine qua non of classic Wilson's disease, does not itself cause the renal pathology, since glomer-

*The mean of the eight patients was probably so remarkably high because the highest concentrations of copper were found in five patients whose deaths were immediately preceded by the sudden release of copper from degenerating hepatocytes and lysed erythrocytes.

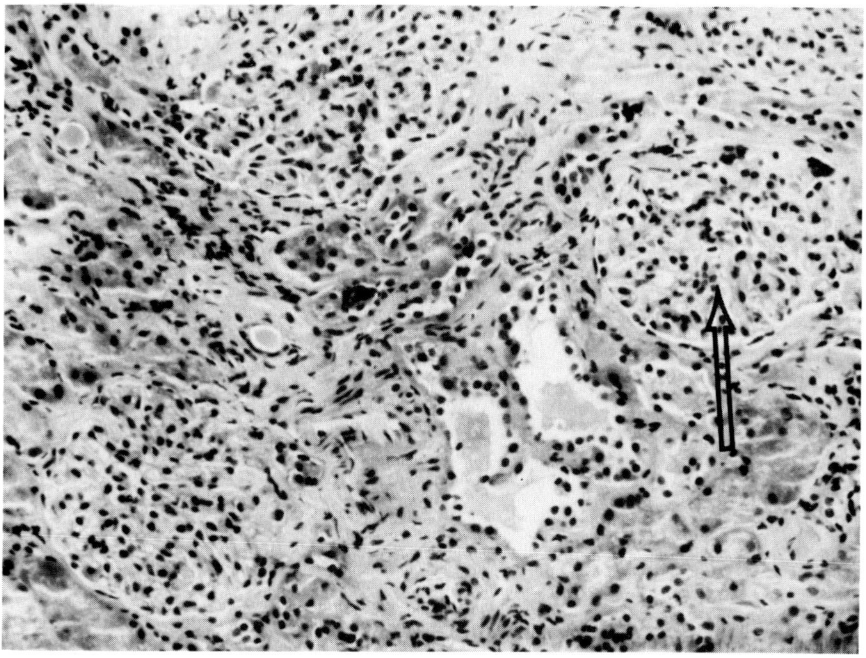

Figure 11–4. Markedly hypercellular glomeruli *(arrow)* in a renal biopsy specimen. Patient I1, with slight neurologic abnormalities but no significant urinary dysfunction. Hematoxylin-eosin. × 160.

ular lesions, the characteristic and nearly sole abnormality in non-Wilsonian cirrhosis,[39] are, as already indicated, rare in Wilson's disease.

CLINICAL PATHOLOGY

The urine of patients with Wilson's disease may contain blood, albumin, glucose, and excessive amounts of phosphate, urate, calcium, bicarbonate, amino acids or peptides.[5, 6, 11–15, 40] Gross hematuria, which is unusual, may occur early in the disease, and it generally disappears completely. We do not know what its relationship (if any) is to the remarkable but apparently asymptomatic glomerular lesions described in the Thai man, in whom hematuria had never been noted. The other abnormalities are probably the consequence of defective proximal tubular function.

Although proximal tubular acidosis, associated with minimal bicarbonate wasting, has been reported in two of 13 patients in one study,[13] defective urinary acidification, occasionally associated with nephrocalcinosis,[10] is more probably due to distal renal tubular acidosis.[9, 10, 13, 14, 35]

In addition to abnormalities in tubular secretory and reabsorptive capacities, Bearn et al.[14] and Leu et al.[35] have demonstrated reductions in renal plasma flow and decreased glomerular filtration rates in patients with advanced Wilson's disease. Impairment of the capacity to concentrate or dilute urine after dehydration or water loading has been noted in a few patients.[35]

CLINICAL EFFECTS

In two of the 151 symptomatic patients whose courses are analyzed in Chapter 14, F8 and L5, gross hematuria was the first clinical manifestation of Wilson's disease. In both, as well as in other reported patients,[41, 42] the hematuria, initially thought to presage glomerulonephritis, ceased spontaneously without progression to chronicity. Microscopic hematuria has been noted in several patients to recur intermittently, and it generally subsides with penicillamine treatment.

When azotemia and electrolyte imbalance accompany severe hepatic insufficiency in patients with Wilson's disease who have not received or responded to decoppering treatment, death is almost inevitable.

The three other effects of Wilsonian renal dysfunction—skeletal abnormalities, renal stones, and acidosis—are rarely clinically significant in untreated patients, in whom the disorders of the central nervous system and liver always predominate. Ironically, as is apparent from Chapter 15, severe proteinuria, the nephrotic syndrome, lupus erythematosus or Goodpasture's syndrome is more likely to occur as a consequence of penicillamine administration than of copper toxicity.

The variety of skeletal effects (described in Chapter 12) are due in part to the hypercalciuria and hyperphosphaturia of the renal lesion.[3, 11, 43]

Renal stones are not uncommon. Seven of 54 patients with Wilson's disease were found to have stones in a study whose authors concluded that abnormalities of acid-base excretion, as well as hypercalciuria (in three of the seven patients), played causal roles.[8] A patient in another study had both renal stones and osteomalacia.[43] The copper concentration in the bladder calculus of one of our patients, T3, was not elevated.

Acidosis is almost always mild and is unlikely to be detected unless a defect in renal acidification is looked for or nephrocalcinosis is seen by x-ray. Except for its synergistic role in forming stones and possibly interfering with the effectiveness of penicillamine therapy,[40] the acidosis of Wilson's disease is not clinically noteworthy.

REFERENCES

1. Mandelbrote, B. M., Stanier, M. W., Thompson, R. H. S., and Thruston, M. N.: Studies on copper metabolism in demyelinating diseases of the central nervous system. Brain *71*:212–228, 1948.
2. Uzman, L., and Denny-Brown, D.: Amino-aciduria in hepato-lenticular degeneration (Wilson's disease). Amer. J. Med. Sci. *215*:599-611, 1948.
3. Cartwright, G. E., Hodges, R. E., Gubler, C. J., Mahoney, J. P., Daum, K., Wintrobe, M. M., and Bean, W. B.: Studies on copper metabolism. XIII. Hepatolenticular degeneration. J. Clin. Invest. *33*:1487-1501, 1954.
4. Hodges, R. E., Kirkendall, W. M., and Gubler, C. J.: Some aspects of kidney function in hepatolenticular degeneration (Wilson's disease). J. Lab. Clin. Med. *47*:337–342, 1956.
5. Asatoor, A. M., Milne, M. D., and Walshe, J. M.: Excretion of peptides and hydroxyproline in Wilson's disease. Clin. Sci. Mol. Med. *51*:369–378, 1976.
6. Asatoor, A. M., Milne, M. D., and Walshe, J. M.: Peptiduria in the Fanconi Syndrome. *In* Peptide Transport and Hydrolysis. Ciba Foundation Symposium 50, Elsevier/North Holland, New York, 1977, pp. 287–298.

7. Stein, W. H., Bearn, A. G., and Moore, S.: The amino acid content of the blood and urine in Wilson's disease. J. Clin. Invest. *33*:410–419, 1953.
8. Wiebers, D. O., Wilson, D. M., McLeod, R. A., and Goldstein, N. P.: Renal stones in Wilson's disease. Amer. J. Med. *67*:249–254, 1979.
9. Cooper, A. M., Eckhardt, R. D., Faloon, W. W., and Davidson, C. S.: Investigation of aminoaciduria in Wilson's disease (hepatolenticular degeneration): Demonstration of a defect of renal function. J. Clin. Invest. *29*:265–278, 1950.
10. Fulop, M., Sternlieb, I., and Scheinberg, I. H.: Defective urinary acidification in Wilson's disease. Ann. Intern. Med. *68*:770–777, 1968.
11. Randall, R. V., Goldstein, N. P., Gross, J. B., and Rosevear, J. W.: Hypercalciuria in hepatolenticular degeneration (Wilson's disease). Amer. J. Med. Sci. *252*:715–720, 1966.
12. Wilson, D. M., and Goldstein, N. P.: Renal urate excretion in patients with Wilson's disease. Kidney Internat. *4*:331–336, 1973.
13. Wilson, D. M., and Goldstein, N. P.: Bicarbonate excretion in Wilson's disease (hepatolenticular degeneration). Mayo Clin. Proc. *49*:394–400, 1974.
14. Bearn, A. G., Yü, T. F., and Gutman, A. B.: Renal function in Wilson's disease. J. Clin. Invest. *36*:1107–1114, 1957.
15. Morgan, H. G., Stewart, W. R., Lowe, K. G., Stowers, J. M., and Johnstone, J. H.: Wilson's disease and the Fanconi syndrome. Quart. J. Med. *31*:361–384, 1962.
16. Forssman, O.: Wilson's disease in a Swedish family. A follow-up study. Acta Med. Scand. *166*:237–239, 1960.
17. Uzman, L. L.: On the relationship of urinary copper excretion to the aminoaciduria in Wilson's disease (hepatolenticular degeneration). Amer. J. Med. Sci. *226*:645–652, 1963.
18. Gilsanz, V., Barrera, A., and Anaya, A.: The renal biopsy in Wilson's disease. Arch. Intern. Med. *105*:758–761, 1960.
19. Canelas, H. M., De Jorge, F. B., Escalante, O. D. and Rocha-Quintao, E. C.: Hepatolenticular degeneration. Clinical and biochemical study of three cases. Arq. Neuro-psiquia. (S. Paulo). *2*:229–250, 1963.
20. Playoust, M. R., and Dale, N. E.: Metabolic balance studies in a patient with Wilson's disease and hypercalciuria. Metabolism *10*:304–314, 1961.
21. Wolff, S. M., and Vanderbilt, M. D.: Renal lesions in Wilson's disease. Lancet *I*:843–845, 1964.
22. Konovalov, N. V.: Gepato-lentikularnaya Degeneraciya. Medgiz, Moscow, 1948.
23. Schaffner, F.: Jaundice, ascites, and corneal discoloration with normal ceruloplasmin. J. Mt. Sinai Hosp. N.Y. *30*:349–360, 1963.
24. McGuire, L. B., and Smith, D. E.: Liver failure in a young man. Va. Med. Month., *95*:218–226, 1968.
25. Yoshitoshi, Y., Oda, T., Yamane, Y., Nagase, M., Mori, K., and Shikata, T.: Renal lesions in Wilson's disease. *In* Wilson's Disease. Birth Defects, Original Article Series, Vol IV. Ed. by Bergsma, D., Scheinberg, I. H., and Sternlieb, I. The National Foundation—March of Dimes, New York, 1968, pp. 104–108.
26. Miller, G. J., and Persaud, V.: Hereditary hepatolenticular degeneration. (Wilson's disease). Report of the first case in Jamaica. Trop. Geogr. Med. *20*:225–232, 1968.
27. Lingaerde, O.: Et tilfelle av hepato-lentikulaer degenerasjon (Hall). Norsk. Mag. Langevidansk. *98*:1267–1282, 1937.
28. Bennet, B., Scheinberg, I. H., and Sternlieb, I.: Unpublished observations.
29. Sherlock, S.: A case of juvenile cirrhosis. Brit. Med. J. *1*:631–637, 1960.
30. Kark, R. M.: Some aspects of nutrition and the kidney. Amer. J. Med. *25*:698–712, 1958.
31. Reynolds, E. S., Tanne, R. L., and Tyler, H. R.: The renal lesion in Wilson's disease. Amer. J. Med. *40*:518–527, 1966.
31a. Gharib, M., Moazzami, R., and Behbakht, Gh: Wilson's disease. Report of a patient with osseous manifestations. Clin. Ped. *9*:625–626, 1970.
32. Hollister, L. E., Cull, V. L., Gonda, V. A., and Kolb, F. O.: Hepatolenticular degeneration. Clinical, biochemical and pathologic study of a patient with fulminant course aggravated by treatment with BAL and versenate. Amer. J. Med. *28*:623–630, 1960.
33. Scheinberg, I. H., and Sternlieb, I.: Metabolism of trace metals. *In* Duncan's Disease of Metabolism. Vol. 2, Endocrinology and Nutrition, 6th ed. Ed. by Bondy, P. K. W. B. Saunders Co., Philadelphia, 1969, pp. 550–564.
34. Walshe, J. M.: Effect of penicillamine on failure of renal acidification in Wilson's disease. Lancet *I*:775–779, 1968.
35. Leu, M. L., Strickland, G. T., and Gutman, R. A.: Renal function in Wilson's disease; response to penicillamine therapy. Amer. J. Med. Sci. *260*:381–398, 1970.
36. Sorenson, L., and Kappas, A.: The effects of penicillamine therapy on uric acid metabolism in Wilson's disease. Trans. Assoc. Amer. Physicians *79*:157–164, 1966.
37. Troelstra, J. A., and Holl, H.: Penicillamine for tubular dysfunction in Wilson's disease. Lancet *I*:1094, 1968.

38. Elsas, L. J., Hayslett, J. P., Spargo, B. H., Durant, J. L., and Rosenberg, L. E.: Wilson's disease with reversible and tubular dysfunction. Correlation with proximal tubular ultrastructure. Ann. Intern. Med. *75*:427–433, 1971.
39. Manigand, G., Taillandier, J., Morel-Maroger, L., and Deparis, M.: La néphropathie glomerulaire des cirrhoses du foie. Ann. Méd. Interne (Paris) *132*:178–182, 1981.
40. Strickland, G. T., and Leu, M.-L.: Wilson's disease. Clinical and laboratory manifestations in 40 patients. Medicine *54*:113–137, 1975.
41. Monnet, P., Gauthier, J., Cotte. J., Vallon, J.-J., Nicholas, A., and Ruitton-Ugliengo: Maladie de Wilson à forme essentielle hépato-renale chez le frère et la soeur et son traitement par la penicillamine. Pédiatrie *16*:565–581, 1961.
42. Pellet, H., Gallard, L., Monier, D., and Ruitton-Ugliengo: Maladie de Wilson's à début trompeur. (Hématurie puis syndrome d'hypertension portale.) Pédiatrie *20*:472–473, 1965.
43. Monro, P.: Effect of treatment on renal function in severe osteomalacia due to Wilson's disease. J. Clin. Pathol. *23*:487–491, 1970.

CHAPTER 12

THE SKELETON AND INTEGUMENT

By 1970 the skeletal changes that had been observed in patients with Wilson's disease included osteoporosis, spontaneous fractures, rickets, osteomalacia, localized demineralization, osteoarthritis, fragmentation of marginal bone, osteochondritis dissecans, osteochondritis of the spine, para-articular calcifications, areas of sclerosis, osseous lacunae and distortions of spinal curvature.[1–3] Psoriatic arthritis developed in one patient of ours, W2.

Over the following decade, chrondromalacia patellae,[4,5] joint hypermobility,[6] polyarthritis[6,7] and intra-articular calcifications[8] have been observed. Although one case of polyarthritis[7] and two of the nine instances of hypermobility reported[6] occurred before penicillamine treatment had been initiated, since the mid-1960s virtually every patient with diagnosed Wilson's disease has been treated with penicillamine, so that most instances of polyarthritis and perhaps some of those of hypermobility may have been due to toxicity of the drug rather than to Wilson's disease.[6]

Comparing the results of skeletal studies performed before and after about 1970 is further complicated: Penicillamine may not only cause osteoarticular disorders in patients with Wilson's disease, but may also prevent rheumatoid arthritis. We know of only two women who suffered from the latter and Wilson's disease—neither has been reported—so that, judging from our experience, the prevalence of patients afflicted with both disorders cannot be much greater than 0.5 per cent, considerably lower than the 2 to 4 per cent of the general population who suffer from rheumatoid arthritis. This disparity may not be statistically significant, because of the rarity of Wilson's disease, and certainly does not prove that penicillamine prevents rheumatoid arthritis, but over the past 20 years the majority of patients with diagnosed and penicillamine-treated Wilson's disease survive beyond middle age, when rheumatoid arthritis commonly begins.[9]

In our series of 38 patients with Wilson's disease,[2] there were only five who showed no bony abnormalities. The rest showed demineralization, and 15 of these showed other abnormalities of bones or joints.

Generalized skeletal demineralization, not radiologically suggestive of osteomalacia, was noted in 21 of 32 consecutive hospital admissions of patients with Wilson's disease who were investigated for osteoarticular lesions.[6] The authors concluded that this demineralization was probably a consequence of hypercalciuria and hyperphosphaturia. Nine of 17 patients showed mild demineralization in another study.[5] Demineralization was seen in intraoral x-ray films of the jawbones of nine of 11 patients with Wilson's disease.[10] Curiously, none of the 11 exhibited evidence of demineralization elsewhere in x-ray surveys of the skeleton. One of the nine showed progressive remineralization in dental x-ray films taken annually for three years after penicillamine therapy (which resulted in marked improvement of her Wilson's disease) was initiated. It is often difficult to determine whether the cause of demineralization, diagnosed on the basis of increased radiolucency, is osteomalacia or osteoporosis,[2, 6] since these can be differentiated with certainty only by histologic and chemical analyses of bone.[11]

In Scotland,[12] India,[13, 14] and Iran[15] seven children with Wilson's disease, aged 7 to 13 years, presented initially with vitamin D–resistant rickets. Malnutrition, severe in at least three of these patients, probably played a synergistic role with hypercalciuria and hyperphosphaturia in causing these instances of rickets, a rare accompaniment of Wilson's disease in the West.

The joint disorders of Wilson's disease are more likely to affect the knees and wrists than other joints. Pain or stiffness in the knees was a complaint of 10 of the 32 patients Golding and Walshe studied,[6] and of six of 14 patients reported by Aksoy and co-workers.[16] Osteochondritis dissecans, chondromalacia patellae, loose bodies, and/or premature degenerative arthritis were noted in knees and wrists of the majority of the 82 patients surveyed in the five major studies of skeletal disorders in Wilson's disease published since 1972.[4–6, 8, 16] In a radiologic and scintigraphic (using ^{99m}technetium) study of 25 penicillamine-treated patients with Wilson's disease (in which 22 patients showed radiologic findings that were interpreted as osteoporosis), the scintigraphic findings showed postinflammatory degenerative changes in 15 joints of eight patients, and synovitis in 22 joints of 10 patients.[17] The polyarthritis of a 14-year-old Iraqi boy, the association of which with Wilson's disease may have been coincidental, affected his knees and elbows.[7]

Conclusive evidence is lacking as to whether copper toxicity is the *direct* cause of any of the skeletal disturbances that have been described in Wilson's disease. The only data compatible with an etiologic role for copper in these abnormalities are analyses of bone and cartilage for copper that have been carried out in two patients with Wilson's disease and two control subjects (Table 12–1).[18] These results suggest there is

TABLE 12–1. Concentration of Copper in Bone and Cartilage (micrograms copper/gram wet tissue)

Tissue	WD 1	WD 2	Control 1	Control 2
Bone	5.5	0.7	0.8	1.7
Cartilage	1.5	2.1	0.7	0.4

considerably more copper than normal in the bone and cartilage of patients with Wilson's disease, particularly since patient WD2 received sufficient penicillamine for four months before death to establish a negative copper balance, whereas patient WD1 had received only BAL for four months, and no decoppering medication for a year before death.

Tending to exculpate copper are the facts that hypercalciuria and hyperphosphaturia (see Chapter 11) must be a major (if not the only) cause of rickets, osteomalacia or demineralization[6, 14]; and that dystonic contractures, immobilization,[6] or chronic liver disease,[11] of whatever etiology, have been shown to cause osteoporosis. Moreover, copper could not be stained with rubeanic acid in biopsy samples of synovia taken from the knees of five patients with Wilson's disease and evidence of arthritis in that joint.[4, 5] Furthermore, experimental copper loading of animals does not produce skeletal changes,[2] although copper *deficiency* does.[19–21] Nor do the changes seen in Wilson's disease resemble the skeletal effects of poisoning by other heavy metals, including cadmium, lead, strontium or bismuth.[2] Finally, despite the claim of two groups of authors that both Wilson's disease and hemochromatosis may be associated with pseudogout,[22, 23] Wilsonian skeletal pathology differs in character and in the parts of the skeleton affected from the arthropathy of idiopathic hemochromatosis.[24]

More data will be required before the role copper toxicity may play in causing the skeletal changes in Wilson's disease can be defined.

Brown pigmentation of the skin—most often present on the shins,[25, 26] but sometimes more diffusely[27]—may be a presenting sign in patients with Wilson's disease. Acanthosis nigricans developed in one patient.[28] A most unusual finding is a bluish discoloration of the lunulae of the nails of the fingers, though not of the toes.[29]

Periodontal disease, generally seen in open-mouthed patients,[30] has been attributed to dryness of the oral mucosa.[31]

REFERENCES

1. Finby, N., and Bearn, A. G.: Roentgenographic abnormalities of the skeletal system in Wilson's disease (hepatolenticular degeneration). Amer. J. Roentgenol. *79*:603–611, 1958.
2. Mindelzun, R., Elkin, M., Scheinberg, I. H., and Sternlieb, I.: Skeletal changes in Wilson's disease. A radiological study. Radiology *94*:127–132, 1970.
3. Boudin, G., and Pépin, B.: Osteoarticular changes in hepatolenticular degeneration. *In* Wilson's Disease: Some Current Concepts. Ed. by Walshe, J. M., and Cumings, J. N. Blackwell, Oxford, 1961, pp. 233–236.
4. Kaklamanis, P., and Spengos, M.: Osteoarticular changes and synovial biopsy findings in Wilson's disease. Ann. Rheum. Dis. *32*:422–427, 1973.
5. Feller, E. R., and Schumacher, H. R.: Osteoarticular changes in Wilson's disease. Arthritis Rheum. *15*:259–266, 1972.
6. Golding, D. N., and Walshe, J. M.: Arthropathy of Wilson's disease. Study of clinical and radiological features in 32 patients. Ann. Rheum. Dis. *36*:99–111, 1977.
7. Bakos, S. N.: Polyarthritis associated with Wilson's disease. Arch. Dis. Child. *54*:985, 1979.
8. Perra, L., Giagheddu, M., Spissu, A., Aresu, G., and Rachele, M. G.: Rilievi clinico-radiologici sulle alterazioni osteo-articolari nella malattia di Wilson. Rass. Med. Sarda (Cagliari) *78*:377–406, 1975.
9. Scheinberg, I. H.: Copper penicillaminate for rheumatoid arthritis? J. Rheumatol. (Suppl. 7) *8*:178–179, 1981.
10. Ogle, R. C., Gibilisco, J. A., Goldstein, N. P., and Randall, R. V.: Oral roentgenographic changes in Wilson's disease. J. Lancet *87*:464–466, 1967.
11. Paterson, C. R., and Losowsky, M. S.: The bones in chronic liver disease. Scand. J. Gastroenterol. *2*:293–300, 1967.

12. Morgan, H. G., Stewart, W. K., Lowe, K. G., Stowers, J. M., and Johnstone, J. H.: Wilson's disease and the Fanconi Syndrome. Quart. J. Med. *31*:361–384, 1962.
13. Mehta, R. S., and Shinde, V. A.: Wilson's disease with rickets. Neurology (India) *13*:67–73, 1965.
14. Joshua, G. E.: Hepatolenticular degeneration (Wilson's disease) and rickets in children. Indian J. Med. Res. *61*:1876–1884, 1973.
15. Gharib, M., Moazzami, R., and Behbakht, G. H.: Wilson's disease. Report of patient with osseous manifestations. Clin. Pediat. *9*:625–626, 1970.
16. Aksoy, M., Camli, N., Dilsen, G., Kocak, N., Erdem, S., Ozdogan, E., Dincol, K., and Dincol, G.: Osteoarticular pains and changes in Wilson's disease. A radiological study in fourteen patients in nine Turkish families. Acta Hepato-Gastroenterol. *22*:164–170, 1975.
17. Canelas, H. M., Carvalho, N., Scaff, M., Vitule, A., Barbosa, E. R., and Azevedo, E. M.: Osteoarthropathy of hepatolenticular degeneration. Acta Neurol. (Scand.) *57*:481–487, 1978.
18. Tu, J.-B., Blackwell, R. Q., and Hou, T.-Y.: Tissue copper levels in Chinese patients with Wilson's disease. Neurology *13*:155–159, 1963.
19. Underwood, E. J.: Trace Elements in Human and Animal Nutrition. Academic Press, New York, 1971, pp. 57–115.
20. Guggenheim, K.: Copper and bones. Isr. J. Med. Sci. *3*:773–775, 1967.
21. Baxter, J. H., and van Wyk, J. H.: Bone disorder associated with copper deficiency; gross morphological, roentgenological and chemical observations. Bull. Johns Hopkins Hosp. *93*:1–23, 1953.
22. Boudin, G., Pépin, B., and Hubault, A.: Les arthropathies de la maladie de Wilson. Rev. Rhum. *31*:594–598, 1964.
23. McCarty, D. J., Pepe, P. F., Solomon, S. D., and Cobb, J.: Inhibition of human erythrocyte pyrophosphatase activity by calcium, cupric and ferrous ions. Arthritis Rheum. *13*:336, 1970.
24. Hamilton, E., Williams, R., Barlow, K. A., and Smith, P. M.: The arthropathy of idiopathic haemochromatosis. Quart. J. Med. *37*:171–182, 1968.
25. Leu, M. L., Strickland, G. T., Wang, C. C., and Chen, T. S. N.: Skin pigmentation in Wilson's disease. J. Amer. Med. Assoc. *211*:1542–1543, 1970.
26. Steiner, P., Frey, P., Lupi, G. A., and Kistler, H. J.: Familliärer Morbus Wilson: Kupferinduzierte Hämolyse, Hyperspleniesyndrom und Hyperpigmentation als Leitsymptome. Schweiz. Med. Wschr. *105*:872–879, 1975.
27. Boudin, G., Pépin, B., Barbizet, J., and Lanièce, M.: Un cas de forme pseudo-sclérose de Westphal-Strumpell. Etude clinique et biologique. Bull. Mém. Soc. Méd. Hôp. Paris. *22*:762, 1957.
28. Ezzo, J. A., Rowley, J. F., and Finnegan, J. V.: Hepatolenticular degeneration associated with acanthosis nigricans. Arch. Int. Med. *100*:827–832, 1957.
29. Bearn, A. G., and McKusick, V. A.: Azure lunulae. An unusual change in the fingernails in two patients with hepatolenticular degeneration (Wilson's disease). J. Amer. Med. Assoc. *166*:904–906, 1958.
30. Tsuha, M., Yamamoto, H., and Urago, A.: Pathohistological report of periodontosis in an autopsy case of Wilson's disease. Nippon Shishubyo Gakkai Kaishi. *22*:130–136, 1980.
31. Stevens, J. B., and Wilkinson, E. G.: Drugs, dry mouth, and dental disease. Psychosomatics *12*:310–311, 1971.

CHAPTER 13

THE HEART AND THE PANCREAS

The effects of Wilson's disease on the heart and pancreas are considered in one chapter. It is curious, as we shall see, that the toxic effects of copper on the heart and pancreas in Wilson's disease are rarely, if ever, of clinical significance, in contrast to those of iron in hemochromatosis.[1, 2]

THE HEART

Although serious cardiac disease is absent in Wilson's disease, several publications describe histologic and ultrastructural changes in the hearts of patients. None, however, describes any definite clinical cardiac dysfunction that can be attributed to copper toxicity.[3–7] Cardiac deaths have occurred in two patients with Wilson's disease—one with ventricular fibrillation, and the other with congestive failure—although there was no increase in cardiac copper or pathologic abnormality found in the first patient at autopsy, and autopsy was not performed on the second.[7a]

In a study of nine patients with Wilson's disease we found five hearts to be hypertrophied, with weights in excess of 350 grams.[8] Histologically, three abnormalities were noted. Both interstitial fibrosis and varying degrees of sclerosis of intramyocardial small vessels were seen in all nine patients. Third, focal, interstitial or perivascular myocarditis was noted in seven patients. In one man, W3, there was fibrosis with mast cells and degenerative changes in a section from the atrioventricular node.

Table 13–1 shows that fibrosis, small-vessel changes and myocardial inflammation (present in W3) were associated with a normal concentration of cardiac copper, whereas in A2, with the highest concentration of copper, no myocardial inflammation was noted. Since mild interstitial or vascular sclerosis was seen in all three age-matched control patients—each with significant hepatic fibrosis or cirrhosis—it is unlikely that the myocardial changes seen in the patients with Wilson's disease were a result of copper toxicity.

TABLE 13–1. Cardiac Pathology and Copper Concentration in Wilson's Disease

CASE	HEART WEIGHT (GRAMS)	INTERSTITIAL FIBROSIS	SMALL-VESSEL PATHOLOGY	MYOCARDIAL INFLAMMATION	COPPER CONCENTRATION* (mcg/gdw)
G1	400	+	+	+	18
A1	200	+	+	+	79
B4	400	+	+	+	228
W3	375	+	+	+	14
A2	350	+	+	−	1348
P1	320	+	+	+	143
S17	450	+	+	+	84
LF (M.G.H.)†	220	+	+	−	21
M2	320	+	+	+	16
Control 1	260	−	+	−	N.A.‡
Control 2	340	−	+	−	N.A.‡
Control 3	290	+	−	−	N.A.‡

*The cardiac concentration of copper of normal subjects has been given as a mean of 16.5 mcg/gdw;[9] as a range of 13.6 to 21.6 mcg/gdw determined in five control subjects;[10] and as a mean of 10.8 mcg/gdw in three control subjects with a range of 10.4 to 15.2 mcg/gdw.[16]

†Massachusetts General Hospital case.

‡Copper analyses were not performed on the control hearts.

The nodal degeneration in W3—a man who died suddenly at age 29, almost certainly because of a cardiac arrhythmia—was probably unrelated to his Wilson's disease. He suffered from sporadic episodes of tachycardia beginning in his fifth year, an age at which *no* clinical effects of copper toxicity are seen in Wilson's disease. Moreover, his myocardial concentration of copper was 14 mcg/gdw, a normal value.

Our data, though limited, do not provide evidence that the pathologic changes seen in the heart in Wilson's disease are proportional to the cardiac concentrations of copper.

Since patients A1 and P1 had been treated with penicillamine for only three days and less than two months, respectively, before death, the cardiac changes seen can hardly be attributed to this drug.

THE PANCREAS

There are no reports of histopathologic changes of the pancreas in Wilson's disease, though they have only rarely been looked for. Moreover, the organ seems to be one of the few tissues in Wilson's disease in which little if any excess copper is found. Only one of five patients in whom pancreatic copper content was determined had a value outside the normal range of 2.4 to 20 mcg/gdw (mean: 7.4)[9]—an untreated case of Plooij et al., with approximately 29 mcg/gdw.[10] Single untreated patients with normal values have been reported by Cartwright et al., 4.2 mcg/gdw;[11]

and Bickel et al., 13.5 mcg/gdw.[12] Two of our treated patients had 0.7 and 4.6 mcg/gdw.

Impaired venous drainage, associated with the patients' portal hypertension, was thought to be the likely cause of diffuse pancreatic enlargement demonstrated ultrasonically in two patients with Wilson's disease.[12a]

Pancreatic dysfunction in Wilson's disease has been investigated by three groups of investigators. Measuring the effects of administering both secretin and pancreozymin to five patients, Lankisch et al.[13] found all to have normal pancreatic secretion. Using the same tests in three patients, Osswald and Niessen[14] found all three to have deficient pancreatic secretion.

Dreiling and Grateron[15] have determined the effect of secretin on four indices of pancreatic function—volume, maximum bicarbonate concentration, amylase secretion and biliary response—in ten patients. Four patients had never received penicillamine before testing; three of these had at least three indices of abnormal function, whereas one secreted greater than normal volume. Of the six treated patients, three exhibited essentially normal function, two were abnormal and one was borderline. But none of the patients had any indication of clinical abnormality.

We know of only one instance in which clinical manifestations of pancreatic disturbance may possibly have been caused by Wilson's disease. A patient of ours, S1, has had recurrent episodes of chronic pancreatitis, without cholelithiasis, over a 13-year period of successful penicillamine treatment that abolished his presenting minimal neurologic and psychiatric disturbances.

REFERENCES

1. Nicholas, G., Bouhour, J. B., Delajartre, A., Goldin, J. F., and Horeau, J.: Myocardiopathie secondaire à l'hémochromatose idiopathique, Quatre observations anatomo-cliniques avec étude du myocarde en microscopie électronique. Arch. Mal. Coeur *64*:1533–1546, 1971.
2. Buja, L. M., and Roberts, W. C.: Iron in the heart. Etiology and clinical significance. Amer. J. Med. *51*:209–221, 1971.
3. Azevedo, E. M., Scaff, M., Barbosa, E. R., Gouveia Neto, A. E., and Canelas, H. M.: Heart involvement in hepatolenticular degeneration. Acta Neurol. Scand. *58*:296–303, 1978.
4. Kaduk, B., Metze, K., Schmidt, P.-F., and Brandt, G.: Secondary athrocytotic cardiomyopathy—heart damage due to Wilson's disease. Virch. Arch. A. Pathol. Anat. Histol. *387*:67–80, 1980.
5. Butt, E. M., Nussbaum, R. E., Gilmour, T. C., and Didio, S. L.: Trace metal patterns in disease states. II. Copper storage diseases, with consideration of juvenile cirrhosis, Wilson's disease, and hepatic copper of the newborn. Amer. J. Clin. Pathol. *30*:479–497, 1958.
6. Bottiger, L. E., and Mollerberg, H.: Increased copper content of hypertrophic myocardium. Acta Med. Scand. *165*:413–416, 1959.
7. Brandt, G.: Zur Diagnose der abdominellen Form des Morbus Wilson. Dtsch. Med. Wschr. *97*:2006–2009, 1972.

7a. Kuan, P.: Fatal cardiac complications of Wilson's disease. Amer. Heart J. *104*:314–316, 1982.

8. Factor, S. M., Cho, S., Sternlieb, I., Scheinberg, I. H., and Goldfischer, S.: The cardiomyopathy of Wilson's disease: Myocardial alterations in nine cases. Virch. Arch. A. Pathol. Anat. *397*:301–311, 1982.
9. Committee on Medical and Biological Effects of Environmental Pollutants.: Human Copper Metabolism. *In* Copper. National Academy of Sciences, Washington, D.C., 1977.
10. Plooij, M., van der Meer, J., and Kaag, A.: Het kopergehalte van endele organen bij een lijder aan de ziekte van Wilson. Ned. Tijdschr. Geneesk. *104*:324–326, 1960.
11. Cartwright, G. E., Hodges, R. E., Gubler, C. J., Mahoney, J. P., Daum, K., Wintrobe, M. M., and Bean, W. B.: Studies on copper metabolism. XIII. Hepatolenticular degeneration. J. Clin. Invest. *33*:1487–1501, 1954.

12. Bickel, H., Neale, F. C., and Hall, G.: A clinical and biochemical study of hepatolenticular degeneration. (Wilson's disease). Quart. J. Med. *25*:527–558, 1957.
12a. Minns, R. A., Eden, O. B., and Hendry, G. M. A.: Pancreatic enlargement and Wilson's disease. Lancet *II*:337–338, 1982.
13. Lankisch, P. G., Kaboth, U., and Koop, H.: Pankreasbeteiligung bei Morbus Wilson? Klin. Wschr. *56*:969–971, 1978.
14. Osswald, P., and Niessen, K. H.: Exokrine Pankreasinsuffizienz bei Morbus Wilson. Klin. Wschr. *54*:839–843, 1976.
15. Dreiling, D. A., and Grateron, H.: Studies in pancreatic secretion VI. The pancreatic function in patients with Wilson's disease. J. Mt. Sinai Hosp. (In Press.)
16. Tu, J.-B., Blackwell, R. Q., and Hou, T.-Y.: Tissue copper levels in Chinese patients with Wilson's disease. Neurology *13*:155–159, 1963.

CHAPTER 14

DIAGNOSIS

Since a physician seeing three new patients every day is unlikely to see more than one patient with Wilson's disease in a 40-year career almost anywhere on earth,[1–3] he can be expected to make the correct health- and life-saving diagnosis in that patient[4] only if he is aware of the protean manifestations of the disorder. "Correct diagnosis inevitably rests on the ability of the clinician to suspect Wilson's disease on a basis of clinical skills."[5] Although patients may be asymptomatic for as long as 40 years, once symptoms or signs of the disease have appeared progression to irreversible pathologic changes or death may occur in a matter of a week or two. A suspected diagnosis should therefore be made or excluded without delay.

The criteria required to confirm or rule out the diagnosis accurately and efficiently vary with the patient's symptomatology or the reason for which he consulted the physician. It will therefore be most helpful to describe the essential diagnostic methodology and indicate precisely how its components are to be applied to patients with different modes of presentation. Figure 14–1 depicts the latter, as a function of age, in 151 patients. When first seen by a physician 30 of these patients manifested symptoms or signs of two of the six varieties of onset shown. Reflecting the sequence of events in the pathogenesis of Wilson's disease, a hepatic onset occurred in 68 patients, only three of whom (5%) were over 20 years of age. In contrast, of 85 patients manifesting initial neurologic or psychiatric disturbance, 33 (39%) were over 20.

DIAGNOSTIC METHODOLOGY

Table 14–1 lists and describes the one examination, *A*, and the four analyses, *B–E*, that are essential to the diagnosis of Wilson's disease. Since it is unusual for any to be done routinely by physicians or clinical laboratories not continually involved in the diagnosis of these patients, the data may not always be reliable unless the following precautions are taken.

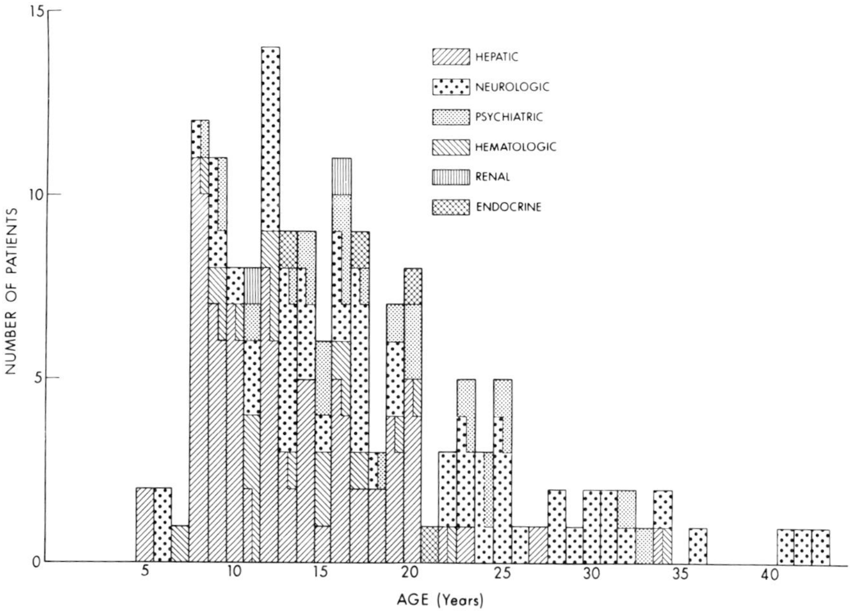

Figure 14–1. Initial mode of clinical onset of Wilson's disease as a function of age. The bars referring to patients presenting with two modes are divided into vertical halves.

A. Corneal examination for Kayser-Fleischer rings must be carried out by an ophthalmologist using a slit-lamp for an unequivocal determination of their presence or absence. There is no value whatever to a statement that is less than certain on this point.

B, C, D. It is unwise to rely on analytic results obtained in a laboratory where only several determinations are made yearly. Too often, and occasionally tragically, such quantitative measurements of the concentrations of ceruloplasmin in serum and of copper in a hepatic biopsy sample or urine have been inaccurate enough to lead to false positive or false negative diagnoses of Wilson's disease.

C. When liver biopsy is performed as a diagnostic procedure, both quantitative determination of the hepatic copper concentration and light microscopic analysis of the sample must be performed. A disposable needle made entirely of steel or a Menghini needle washed with EDTA and rinsed with demineralized water should be used. The propellant solution should be 5 per cent dextrose in water (not saline, which will dissolve sufficient copper from the brass in a Menghini needle to contaminate the sample grossly). Two cores of liver should be obtained. In addition to tissue for histology, about 10 to 15 mg of wet liver is required to determine the hepatic copper concentration accurately.

D. Urinary collections must be made in copper-free vessels with precautions against contamination. None of a number of investigations using the administration of penicillamine to increase urinary copper excretion has yielded a diagnostic index clearly superior to the simple measurement of spontaneous 24-hour excretion. Thus, there was little

TABLE 14–1. The Essential Diagnostic Indices of Wilson's Disease (WD)

Index	Characteristic Positive Value in WD	Conditions with Possible False Positive Results	Conditions with Possible False Negative Results	Notes
A. Kayser-Fleischer rings	Present	Primary biliary cirrhosis	Early Wilson's disease	See text and Ch. 10
B. Ceruloplasmin in serum	<20 mg/dl	Protein loss; kwashiorkor; marasmus; severe copper deficiency; hereditary hypoceruloplasminemia; WD heterozygosity; fulminant hepatitis; Menkes' syndrome	5% of WD patients; any WD patient if pregnant, receiving estrogens, or with acute (including hepatic) inflammation or neoplasm	See Ch. 3
C. Hepatic copper concentration	>250 mcg/gdw	Primary biliary cirrhosis; cholestatic syndromes; Indian childhood cirrhosis	Treated WD	Histology of biopsy sample essential See Ch. 5
D. 24-hour urinary copper	>100 mcg	Concurrent penicillamine, BAL, or Trien administration; chronic hepatitis; cirrhosis; cholestatic or nephrotic syndrome	Treated WD	See text
E. Radiocopper incorporation into ceruloplasmin	Very low	Ceruloplasmin <20 mg/dl; WD heterozygosity	Pregnancy; estrogens; inflammation or neoplasia in Wilson's disease	See text

difference in the overlap in the ranges of copper excreted by patients with Wilson's disease or by those with cholestasis, hepatitis or cirrhosis, whether or not the subjects were given 10 mg penicillamine/kg body weight.[6] Paradoxically, in another study, following the administration of 0.5 g penicillamine, 18 patients with non-Wilsonian neurologic disease excreted, on average, over twice as much radiocopper as did nine asymptomatic patients with Wilson's disease.[7] In a third investigation, in which 12 subjects received 1.0 g of penicillamine, although there was no overlap in total copper excreted by three patients with Wilson's disease compared with seven control subjects and two patients with cirrhosis,[8] there *was* overlap of the amount of copper excreted by the patients with Wilson's disease compared with that excreted by patients with hepatitis and cholestasis receiving *less* penicillamine (10 mg/kg body weight),[6] as well as with that excreted by four control subjects and six patients with chronic active liver disease receiving *more* penicillamine (1.5 g).[9]

E. The determination of the rate of incorporation of radiocopper into ceruloplasmin must be carried out in an arbitrarily standardized manner and in a large enough number of patients with Wilson's disease, heterozygotes and various controls[10] to be of statistical significance. The procedure we devised more than 20 years ago,[11] primarily to detect heterozygous carriers of the WD gene, is simple and reliable and has since proven capable of sharply distinguishing patients with Wilson's

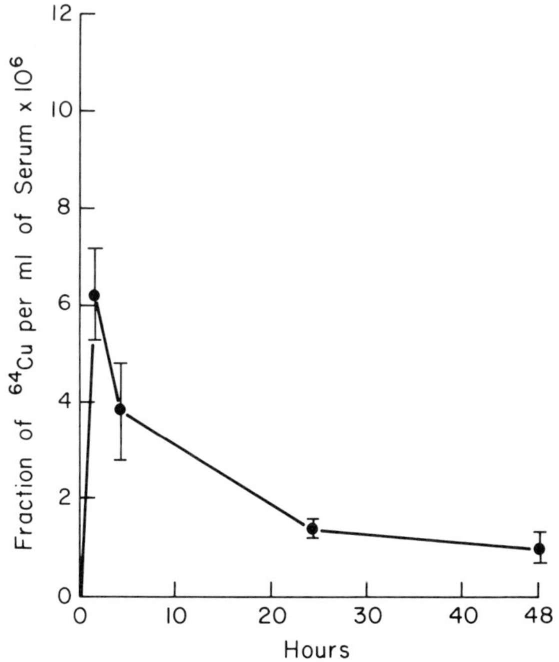

Figure 14–2. Mean (±SEM) concentrations of ^{64}Cu in serum of 11 patients with Wilson's disease and serum ceruloplasmin concentrations ranging from 16.6 to 29.3 mg/dl at intervals following ingestion of 2.0 mg. of radiocopper. (Reprinted from Gastroenterology 77:138–142, 1979, with permission. Copyright 1979 by the American Gastroenterological Association.)

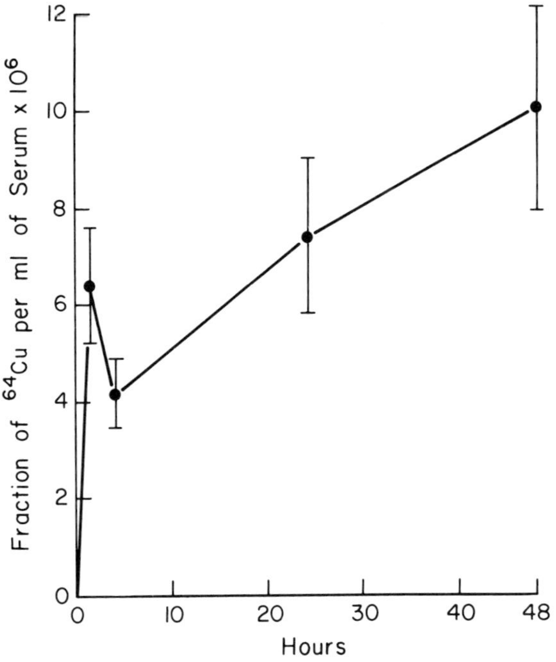

Figure 14–3. Mean (±SEM) concentrations of ^{64}Cu in serum of 11 patients with miscellaneous liver diseases and serum ceruloplasmin concentrations ranging from 24.5 to 58.4 mg/dl at intervals following ingestion of 2.0 mg of radiocopper. (Reprinted from Gastroenterology *77*:138–142, 1979, with permission. Copyright 1979 by the American Gastroenterological Association.)

disease from normal homozygotes with liver disease.[12] A dose of 2.0 mg of radiocopper, as the sulfate or acetate, containing about 0.3 to 0.5 mCi ^{64}Cu is administered in about 100 to 150 ml of fruit juice or ginger ale (*not* in milk) following a fast of at least eight hours. The concentration of ^{64}Cu in serum is determined 1, 2, 4, 24 and 48 hours after its ingestion. In any subject the concentration of ^{64}Cu reaches an initial maximum in the 1- or 2-hour serum sample and then falls. Within the next two to four hours, in individuals without Wilson's disease, the serum concentration of ^{64}Cu rises again (as the radiocopper is incorporated into ceruloplasmin), to approach or exceed, in the 24- or 48-hour sample, the initial maximum. In patients with Wilson's disease, this secondary rise in the serum concentration of ^{64}Cu is absent *even in the presence of a normal ceruloplasmin concentration* (Figs. 14–2 and 14–3).

DIAGNOSIS OF PATIENTS PRESENTING WITH NEUROLOGIC DISEASE

Together with brief descriptions of a number of exemplary patients, the various modes of neurologic onset are set forth in Chapter 8. In any such patient corneal slit-lamp examination and the determination of the serum ceruloplasmin concentration should be carried out as soon as feasible; the absence of Kayser-Fleischer rings excludes the diagnosis, only provided that the patient has not received more than a few weeks of treatment with penicillamine, trien or BAL.

If the serum ceruloplasmin is <20 mg/dl, the diagnosis of Wilson's disease is probable. But before treatment is begun, Kayser-Fleischer rings *must* be proven to be present; a patient *with* neurologic disease and *without* rings (who has not been "decoppered") does *not* have Wilson's disease.

If Kayser-Fleischer rings are present and the serum ceruloplasmin is >20mg/dl, the diagnosis should be confirmed by the results of a hepatic biopsy or a radiocopper incorporation test.

DIAGNOSIS OF PATIENTS PRESENTING WITH PSYCHIATRIC DISEASE

In at least 10 per cent of symptomatic patients, the first clinical manifestation of Wilson's disease is psychiatric. With one or more of the disturbances described in Chapter 9, a patient may seek psychiatric help or may be brought to a physician by a relative.

If there is a family history of Wilson's disease, or particularly in the young, if the psychiatrist is not quite certain what disorder the psychodynamics of the clinical picture represent, the ceruloplasmin concentration should be determined. This is an inexpensive and risk-free procedure, and in at least one major psychiatric center in the United States routine measurement of ceruloplasmin is made on almost every inpatient. In the overwhelming majority of patients, the ceruloplasmin will be >20 mg/dl, making the diagnosis of Wilson's disease very unlikely. If it is <20 mg/dl, or if the physician is uneasy despite a ceruloplasmin of >20 mg/dl, corneal slit-lamp examination is indicated. With almost as much certainty as in the untreated neurologically affected patient, the presence of Kayser-Fleischer rings confirms, and the absence excludes, the diagnosis of Wilson's disease. In the presence of rings *and* a ceruloplasmin of >20 mg/dl, hepatic biopsy or a measure of radiocopper incorporation into ceruloplasmin should be shown to be characteristic of Wilson's disease before the commitment to lifelong treatment with pencillamine is made.

DIAGNOSIS OF PATIENTS PRESENTING WITH LIVER DISEASE

Liver disease, first manifest between the ages of 5 and 35 years,[13] may, as discussed in Chapter 7, be Wilson's disease presenting as acute hepatitis,[13] fulminant hepatitis,[13, 13a] chronic active hepatitis[13–15] or cirrhosis.[13] (If either of the first two is accompanied by hemolytic anemia, the diagnosis of Wilson's disease is more likely than any other.) This mode of presentation may be masked as an endocrine disturbance (menstrual irregularities, repeated miscarriages, or delayed puberty), a probable consequence of liver disease; or as a hematologic abnormality, with bleeding, bruising, leukopenia or thrombocytopenia.

Because ceruloplasmin is synthesized in the liver and is an acute-phase reactant, and because the excretion of copper in individuals *without* Wilson's disease is dependent on normal biliary secretion, the diagnosis of patients with hepatic onset is more difficult than that of patients whose clinical illness begins neurologically or psychiatrically. In the latter two cases, a determination of serum ceruloplasmin and a corneal slit-lamp examination will almost always suffice diagnostically, but a correct diagnosis of Wilson's disease may be missed in the patient with hepatic presentation if only these two indices are evaluated. A concentration of ceruloplasmin that has been diagnostically low for years of symptomless Wilson's disease may be raised into the normal range by the copper-caused active liver disease that has finally become manifest. And Kayser-Fleischer rings are understandably and frequently absent in these patients, who, by definition, have manifested no signs or symptoms of copper toxicity in any extrahepatic site.

Reliance on a ceruloplasmin determination or a slit-lamp examination alone can be almost equally calamitous in leading to a false positive diagnosis of Wilson's disease. A ceruloplasmin of <20 mg/dl may be found in a patient with non-Wilsonian fulminant hepatitis whose dying liver is unable to synthesize normal amounts of ceruloplasmin. And Kayser-Fleischer rings may be present in a patient with primary biliary cirrhosis or other cholestatic syndrome (see Chapter 10).

If the serum ceruloplasmin concentration is <20 mg/dl and Kayser-Fleischer rings are present, the diagnosis of Wilson's disease is certain. The 24-hour urinary copper excretion will generally be >100 mcg, unless the patient has received appreciable penicillamine therapy. Nevertheless, although not necessary for diagnosis in this situation, a hepatic biopsy is helpful in the management of the patient, unless it is precluded by clotting abnormalities. And, if, in the presence of a ceruloplasmin concentration of <20 mg/dl, slit-lamp examination and urinary copper excretion do not lead to an unequivocal confirmation or exclusion of Wilson's disease, a hepatic biopsy *must* be performed sooner or later, since a measurement of radiocopper incorporation is of no value in the face of ceruloplasmin deficiency.

If the ceruloplasmin concentration is >20 mg/dl, but <30 mg/dl, the diagnosis of Wilson's disease is by no means excluded, as is apparent from Table 14–1 and Chapter 3. Particularly if there is a positive family history or persistent transaminasemia (note reference 16 and patient F9), a liver biopsy and slit-lamp examination should be performed. The presence of Kayser-Fleischer rings makes the diagnosis probable despite the fact that these may be seen in primary biliary cirrhosis or cholestatic syndromes, since, in these disorders rings are almost always accompanied by a ceruloplasmin concentration of >30 mg/dl.

At a time when we were insufficiently aware of the difficulties in diagnosing Wilson's disease in a patient with hepatic onset, we concurred in an erroneous diagnosis of this illness in a patient who had already received a liver transplant.[17] Hepatic precoma, finely nodular cirrhosis (with a copper concentration of 1313 mcg/g dry liver) and histopathology "consistent with Wilson's disease" misled us in this 11-year-old white boy despite repeated ceruloplasmin concentrations that were between 26 and

31 mg/dl and a 24-hour urinary copper of 50 mcg. Moreover, we disregarded the normal results of radiocopper incorporation tests in both parents that should have indicated to us that there was almost no chance whatever that the boy had Wilson's disease. And, before transplantation (it would have been useless after), that test had not been performed on the patient himself. We could not know, in 1971, that this patient probably suffered from hepatic copper overload of the type thought to be characteristic of Indian childhood cirrhosis and only recently described in white Americans.[18]

DIAGNOSIS OF PATIENTS WITH RENAL ABNORMALITIES

Following the findings, in 1948, of cupriuria in Wilson's disease by Mandelbrote et al.[19] and of aminoaciduria by Uzman and Denny-Brown,[20] other indices of impaired glomerular and tubular renal function were soon discovered. Hematuria, hyperphosphaturia, hypercalciuria, hyperuricosuria, glycosuria and renal tubular acidosis may directly or indirectly (by leading to hypophosphatemia, hypouricemia, renal calculi or nephrocalcinosis) first bring a patient with Wilson's disease to a physician. If a serum ceruloplasmin is >20 mg/dl, Wilson's disease may be excluded unless there is a family history of the illness or no other cause for the manifestation is found. In the latter case, corneal slit-lamp examination, determination of 24-hour urinary copper or liver biopsy may be indicated.

DIAGNOSIS OF ASYMPTOMATIC PATIENTS

There are four groups of subjects in this category.

1. *Blood relatives of a patient with Wilson's disease.* Siblings, who have an a priori chance of one in four of having the disorder, require, at a minimum, a history and general physical examination, with particular attention to the size of the liver and spleen; corneal slit-lamp examination; and ceruloplasmin determination. Other blood relatives probably need only determinations of ceruloplasmin and aminotransferase levels.

If the ceruloplasmin concentration is <20 mg/dl, a hepatic biopsy sample should be obtained despite the fact that the diagnosis of Wilson's disease is certain if Kayser-Fleischer rings are present. Nevertheless, a hepatic copper concentration of >250 mcg/gdw is necessary to confirm the diagnosis and convince the patient and his physician of the certainty of the diagnosis, for the reason given in 3, below.

If the ceruloplasmin concentration is >20 mg/dl, but transaminase levels are increased or enlargement of liver or spleen is present, a liver biopsy and a radiocopper incorporation test should be performed. If transaminases are normal and there is no hepatic or splenic enlargement, Wilson's disease is very unlikely, but the subject should be observed yearly if the propositus exhibited a ceruloplasmin of >20 mg/dl at the time of diagnosis.

2. *Healthy subjects, without Kayser-Fleischer rings, in whom a concentration of ceruloplasmin of <20 mg/dl is found on routine testing or screening.* Based on a worldwide incidence of Wilson's disease of $30/10^6$,[1–3] and a corresponding incidence of WD heterozygotes of 1 in 90 (of whom about 20 per cent have a ceruloplasmin of <20 mg/dl), each of these subjects has about 1 chance in 70 of having Wilson's disease (see Chapter 2). The other 69 subjects are almost certain to be heterozygous carriers of a single Wilson's disease gene.

If transaminase levels are normal and there is no hepatomegaly or splenomegaly, Wilson's disease is unlikely, but the subject should be warned to return to the physician if any relevant symptom or sign should appear.

If transaminase levels are elevated or there is enlargement of spleen or liver, hepatic biopsy must be performed.

3. *Individuals in whom Kayser-Fleischer rings are found on routine ophthalmologic examination.* If the ceruloplasmin concentration is <20 mg/dl, the diagnosis of Wilson's disease is confirmed, *but* (just as mandatorily as when the ceruloplasmin concentration is >20 mg/dl) a liver biopsy must be performed before committing the patient to lifelong therapy. Primarily this is to allay doubts that may arise years later when Kayser-Fleischer rings have disappeared and the patient, in excellent health because of the penicillamine he has taken, may think he no longer needs the drug.

4. *Individuals with unexplained and persistent transaminasemia.* A liver biopsy shoud be performed and urinary copper excretion measured regardless of whether the ceruloplasmin is greater or less than 20 mg/dl.

DIAGNOSTIC PITFALLS

- It may be impossible to make a diagnosis of Wilson's disease, except on the basis of the history, in a patient who has, through long-term treatment with penicillamine, become symptomless and lost his Kayser-Fleischer rings and in whom the concentration of ceruloplasmin is normal.
- Wilson's disease may be erroneously excluded if it is overlooked that a normal concentration of ceruloplasmin, >20 mg/dl, is found in about 5 per cent of patients. (It is, however, very uncommon for a patient with Wilson's disease to have a ceruloplasmin concentration >30 mg/dl.) Moreover, a patient's usual and diagnostically low level may be misleadingly elevated above 20 mg/dl by hepatitis,[13] inflammatory or neoplastic disease, estrogen administration or pregnancy. (See Table 14–1 and Chapter 3.)
- Conversely, if a ceruloplasmin of <20 mg/dl is the only criterion relied upon, Wilson's disease will be falsely diagnosed if it is not recognized, as pointed out above, that there are about 70 times as many heterozygous carriers of one WD gene with <20 mg/dl as hypoceruloplasminemic patients with Wilson's disease. Moreover, ceruloplasmin deficiency may be present in a patient with any disorder associated with severe intestinal or renal protein loss, or in a patient with hereditary hypoceruloplasminemia.[21]

• If it is based on elevations of urinary copper excretion and hepatic copper concentration, a false diagnosis of Wilson's disease may be made in instances of chronic active hepatitis, with or without cirrhosis, cholestatic syndromes or primary biliary cirrhosis.[22] Patients with these conditions may also exhibit Kayser-Fleischer rings as well as hepatic copper concentrations indistinguishable from those seen in Wilson's disease, but they almost always have normal or elevated concentrations of ceruloplasmin and laboratory findings of cholestasis not seen in Wilson's disease. In one study of 54 patients with non-Wilsonian liver disease none had deficiency of ceruloplasmin[22]; two other reports[23, 24] suggest that very rarely non-Wilsonian liver disease that is not fulminant may be associated with deficiency of ceruloplasmin, possibly the coincidental occurrence of such liver disease in a heterozygous carrier of one WD gene.

• Since all newborn infants exhibit deficiency of ceruloplasmin and a hepatic copper concentration that is above normal, it is fruitless to attempt the diagnosis of Wilson's disease before the patient is six months of age.

There are other tests that, though of little specific diagnostic value, may be of use in the clinical management of patients.

1. Abdominal computed tomography (CT) of patients with liver disease (including one with Wilson's disease) in whom increased hepatic copper concentrations were present yielded normal attenuation values. Cranial CT[25a] has revealed hypodensity of the basal ganglia, ventricular dilatation, and cortical and brain stem atrophy in more than 90 per cent of 40 patients with neurologic abnormalities due to Wilson's disease.[26] In three other studies, involving a total of 27 patients with Wilson's disease, hypodensity of the basal ganglia was seen (occasionally with other abnormalities), but in only 63 per cent of patients with neurologic or psychiatric manifestations.[27–29] Williams and Walshe noted correlation of clinical with CT improvement,[26] but one patient of Harik and Post's improved clinically with penicillamine therapy, despite worsening of the CT abnormalities.[29] The greatest value of CT scans in Wilson's disease is probably diagnostic: Just as the incidental discovery of Kayser-Fleischer rings may lead to a diagnosis of otherwise unsuspected Wilson's disease, so may a finding of hypodense basal ganglia in a CT scan.

2. Nuclear magnetic resonance (NMR) imaging of the brain may reveal more details of the intracranial abnormalities than do cranial CT scans in Wilson's disease.[30]

3. Plain abdominal x-ray films may reveal cholelithiasis, nephrolithiasis, nephrocalcinosis (see Fig. 11–1) or splenomegaly.

4. Radioisotope scans with ^{99m}Tc sulfur colloid may demonstrate the size and shape of the liver, nonhomogeneous uptake by the liver or an increased proportion of the colloid in an enlarged spleen or in bone marrow. This procedure is particularly useful in neurologically affected patients who are unable to relax their abdominal musculature to permit satisfactory palpation for the liver or spleen.

5. Esophageal x-ray films, with barium; splenoportography; or arteriography may be useful in patients suspected of having clinically significant portal hypertension as a complication of Wilson's disease.

6. Laparoscopy, for which there is ever little if any clinical justifica-

tion, has permitted visualizing the characteristic appearance of nodular cirrhosis.

7. Electroencephalograms may be of value in patients with seizures.

8. Brainstem auditory evoked responses were abnormal in patients with Wilson's disease and neurologic symptoms, although *normal* responses were seen in those without neurologic involvement as well as in 19 of 20 patients with spinocerebellar degeneration.[31]

9. Psychometric studies may reveal that the manifest behavioral disturbance or psychiatric syndrome is partly, if not wholly, organic in nature; they also may often show the patient to have an I.Q. that is considerably higher than his appearance, dysarthria, or inability to write suggests.

REFERENCES

1. Bachmann, H., Lossner, J., Grub, B., and Ruchholtz, V.: Die Epidemiologie der Wilsonschen Erkrankung in der DDR und die derzeitige Problematik einer populationgenetischen Bearbeitung. Psychiat. Neurol. Med. Psychol. *30*:393–400, 1979.
2. Saito, T.: An assessment of efficiency in potential screening for Wilson's disease. J. Epidemiol. Comm. Health *35*:274–280, 1981.
3. Vital Statistics of the United States. Vol. II, Mortality, Part A, Tables 1–23, 1968–1978; Dr. Harry M. Rosenberg (personal communication).
4. Scheinberg, I. H.: Penicillamine in Wilson's disease. Lancet *I*:1469, 1982.
5. Walshe, J. M.: Wilson's disease. *In* Diseases of the Liver. Ed. by Schiff, L., and Schiff, E. R., J. B. Lippincott, Philadelphia, 1982, pp. 1043–1059.
6. Frommer, D. J.: Urinary copper excretion and hepatic copper concentration in liver disease. Digestion *21*:169–178, 1981.
7. Gibbs, K., Hanka, R., and Walshe, J. M.: The urinary excretion of radiocopper in presymptomatic and symptomatic Wilson's disease, heterozygotes and controls: Its significance in diagnosis and management. Quart. J. Med. *47*:349–364, 1978.
8. Blehova, B., and Heyrovsky, L.: Penicillamine used as a diagnostic aid in hepatolenticular degeneration (Wilson's disease). Czech. Pediatrie *16*:809–811, 1961.
9. Lynch, R. E., Lee, G. R., and Cartwright, G. E.: Penicillamine-induced cupriuria in normal subjects and in patients with active liver disease. Proc. Sco. Exptl. Biol. Med. *142*:128–130. 1973.
10. Vierling, J. M., Shrager, R., Rumble, W. F., Aamodt, R., Berman, M. D., and Jones, E. A.: Incorporation of radiocopper into ceruloplasmin in normal subjects and in patients with primary biliary cirrhosis and Wilson's disease. Gastroenterology *74*:652–660, 1978.
11. Sternlieb, I., Morell, A. G., Bauer, C. D., Combes, B., DeBobes-Sternberg, S., and Scheinberg, I. H.: Detection of the heterozygous carrier of the Wilson's disease gene. J. Clin. Invest. *40*:707–715, 1961.
12. Sternlieb, I., and Scheinberg, I. H.: The role of radiocopper in the diagnosis of Wilson's disease. Gastroenterology *77*:138–142, 1979.
13. Sternlieb, I.: Diagnosis of Wilson's disease. Gastroenterology *74*:787–789, 1978.

13a. McCullough, A. J., Fleming, C. R., Thistle, J. L., Baldus, W. P., Ludwig, J., McCall, J. T., and Dickson, E. R.: Diagnosis of Wilson's disease presenting as fulminant hepatic failure. Gastroenterology *84*:161–167, 1983.

14. Thompson, W. G., St. George Hyslop, P., Barr, R., and Sass-Kortsak, A.: Wilson's disease: a common liver disorder? CMAJ *117*:45–48, 1977.
15. Sternlieb, I., and Scheinberg, I. H.: Chronic hepatitis as a first manifestation of Wilson's disease. Ann. Int. Med. *76*:59–64, 1972.
16. Stillman, A. E., and Rohr, L. R.: Persistant transaminasemia and fatty liver. Amer. J. Dis. Child. *136*:242–244, 1982.
17. Dubois, R. S., Giles, G., Rodgerson, D. O., Lilly, J., Martineau, G., Halgrimson, C. G., Schroter, G., Starzl, T. E., Sternlieb, I., and Scheinberg, I. H.: Orthotopic liver transplantation for Wilson's disease. Lancet *I*:505–508, 1971.
18. Lefkowitch, J. H., Honig, C. L., King, M. E., and Hagstrom, J. W. C.: Hepatic copper overload and features of Indian childhood cirrhosis in an American sibship. N. Engl. J. Med. *307*:271–277, 1982.
19. Mandelbrote, B. M., Stanier, M. W., Thompson, R. H. S., and Thruston, M. N.: Studies on copper metabolism in demyelinating diseases of the central nervous system. Brain *17*:212–228, 1948.
20. Uzman, L., and Denny-Brown, D.: Amino-aciduria in hepatolenticular degeneration (Wilson's disease). Amer. J. Med. Sci. *215*:599–611, 1948.

21. Edwards, C. Q., Williams, D. M., and Cartwright, G. E.: Hereditary hypoceruloplasminemia. Clin. Gen. *15*:311–316, 1979.
22. LaRusso, N. F., Summerskill, W. H., and McCall, J. T.: Abnormalities of chemical tests for copper metabolism in chronic active liver disease: differentiation from Wilson's disease. Gastroenterology *70*:653–655, 1976.
23. Perman, J. A., Werlin, S. L., Grand, R. J., and Watkins, J. B.: Laboratory measures of copper metabolism in the differentiation of chronic active hepatitis and Wilson's disease in children. J. Pediat. *94*:564–568, 1979.
24. Spechler, S. J., and Koff, R. S.: Wilson's disease: diagnostic difficulties in the patient with chronic hepatitis and hypoceruloplasminemia. Gastroenterology *78*:803–806, 1980.
25. Smevik, B., Ritland, S., Nilsen, T., and Johansen, O.: Liver attenuation values at computed tomography related to liver copper content. Scand. J. Gastroenterol. *17*:461–463, 1982.
25a. Seleker, K., Kansu, T., and Zileli, T.: Computed tomography in Wilson's disease. Arch. Neurol. *38*:727–728, 1981.
26. Williams, F. J. B., and Walshe, J. M.: Wilson's disease. An analysis of the cranial computerized tomographic appearances found in 60 patients and the changes in response to treatment with chelating agents. Brain *104*:735–752, 1981.
27. Merland, J.-J., Chiras, J., Melki, J. P., and Cassan, J. L.: Étude tomodensitométrique dans la maladie de Wilson. Neuroradiology *16*:269–270, 1978.
28. Kendall, B. E., Pollock, S. S., Bass, N. M., and Valentine, A. R.: Wilson's disease. Clinical correlation with cranial computed tomography. Neuroradiology *22*:1–5, 1981.
29. Harik, S. I., and Post, J. D.: Computed tomography in Wilson disease. Neurology *31*:107–110, 1981.
30. Lawler, G. A., Pennock, J. M., Steiner, R. E., Jenkins, W. J., Sherlock, S., and Young, I. R.: Nuclear magnetic resonance (NMR) imaging in Wilson's disease. J. Comput. Assist. Tomogr. *7*:1–8, 1983.
31. Fujita, M., Hosaki, M., and Miyazaki, M.: Brainstem auditory evoked responses in spinocerebellar degeneration and Wilson disease. Ann. Neurol. *9*:42–47, 1981.

CHAPTER 15

TREATMENT

Wilson's disease is one of the very few forms of serious hepatic, neurologic or psychiatric disease for which specific, effective pharmacologic therapy is available.[1–9a] In virtually every patient who is asymptomatic, and in many of those who are ill, decoppering therapy can maintain or restore normal health and longevity, despite the genetic abnormality these patients possess.

MANAGEMENT OF THE PATIENT

Treatment, which must begin when (and only when) the diagnosis is certain, consists, in the vast majority of patients, of the daily oral administration of capsules or tablets of D-penicillamine (beta,beta-dimethylcysteine; D-mercaptovaline) for the rest of the patient's life. Except for children under 5 years of age, one gram of penicillamine daily, administered by mouth in four divided doses 30 to 45 minutes before, or two or more hours after eating, constitutes the basic therapeutic regimen. This applies to all patients, whether ill or asymptomatic. In younger children the daily dose of penicillamine should be 0.02 g per kilogram weight rounded to the nearest multiple of 0.25 g.

The importance of taking the drug when there is no food in the stomach has been demonstrated by a study in which considerably less of the administered amount was absorbed when the penicillamine was taken with or soon after meals.[10]

Because of a possible antipyridoxine effect of penicillamine,[11, 12] the patient should also receive 25 mg of pyridoxine daily. A multivitamin preparation that contains no copper may be of value, particularly in growing children who are inadequately nourished or exhibit hepatic dysfunction, but it should be taken with a meal. We have never found it necessary to supplement the diet with zinc or other minerals routinely, although, in menstruating patients, iron supplements may be indicated; these should not be given together with a dose of penicillamine.

When decoppering treatment was first recognized as essential treatment for Wilson's disease the following were generally considered to be important parts of the patient's regimen: a diet low in copper; drinking and cooking with distilled water; and the ingestion of sulfurated potash with meals to precipitate ingested copper in the gastrointestinal tract. None has since proven necessary if the patient takes penicillamine regularly, although it is probably wise for the patient to avoid eating large quantities of liver, chocolate, nuts, mushrooms and shellfish—foods that are particularly rich in copper.[13–15]

For the first month of therapy the patient should be seen by the physician at least once a week (more frequently if the patient is not a reliable observer) because of the possibility of early toxic reactions to penicillamine. The patient's temperature should be taken every night; white blood cell, differential and platelet counts done thrice weekly; and routine urinalysis performed weekly. If all has gone well, the physician can see the patient less often, but at least once a month during the first year of treatment.

In about 10 per cent of patients with neurologic manifestations, these may worsen during the first weeks or months of penicillamine therapy. The patient must be warned of this possibility *before* treatment begins in order to avoid his abandoning penicillamine in dismay. What causes such a response to penicillamine—paradoxical, since it generally occurs in the face of an adequately increased urinary excretion of copper—is unknown. Continued administration of the drug or *temporary* interruption of treatment is almost always followed by steady improvement.

The patient's clinical course will determine how many of the following criteria for assessing the effectiveness and safety of treatment are to be carried out at each visit: interval history; physical, neurologic and corneal examination; complete blood cell and platelet counts; urinalysis; liver tests; and analyses of serum for ceruloplasmin, and copper, and of an aliquot of a 24-hour urine collection for copper. Patients must be encouraged to contact their physicians at the slightest suspicion of any symptom or sign of Wilson's disease or penicillamine toxicity, about both of which they should be appropriately aware.

At each visit the physician should afford the patient an opportunity to talk freely, permitting evaluation of both the patient's psychiatric and physical state. The skin should be observed for signs of penicillamine toxicity, jaundice, bruising or spider angiomata. The abdomen should be examined to assess liver and spleen size and the presence or absence of ascites, if the latter has been a problem. Neurologic examination can be limited to those functions affected by Wilson's disease, with emphasis on those known to have been involved in the patient. Handwriting samples can often provide simple and dramatic documentation of improvement.

We have found the value of the physical examination to be enhanced if a trained observer—an ophthalmologist—performs slit-lamp examination of the cornea and describes semiquantitatively the state of the Kayser-Fleischer rings at intervals of approximately one year. The intensity and appearance of the rings; the fractions of the vertical and horizontal corneal radii they encroach upon; and, if they are not completely circumferential, the degrees of arc involved by the crescents should be noted and recorded.

Fading or disappearance of rings or crescents is a valuable objective sign that copper is being removed from the patient,[16–19] but this cannot be used to monitor therapy. The persistence of rings in the face of a good clinical response—not uncommon in patients who are over 25 or 30 years old when first treated—is not a cause for concern, but the reappearance or intensification of crescents or rings strongly suggests that the patient is no longer taking his penicillamine in adequate dosage.

The serum should be analyzed quantitatively by a reliable laboratory for ceruloplasmin and copper, at intervals of one or two months during the first six to twelve months of treatment and once or twice yearly thereafter if the patient is doing well. These two measurements provide the best indication of whether the dose of penicillamine actually being taken by the patient is adequate, since they permit calculation of the concentration of the free, diffusible fraction of serum copper that is the ultimate cause of the disease. Free copper—the difference between total serum copper and ceruloplasmin-bound copper—is less than 10 mcg/dl of serum in adequately treated patients as well as in most normal individuals. In untreated or inadequately treated patients, free copper is generally considerably greater than 10 mcg/dl, and may exceed 50 mcg/dl. Obviously, for the calculated value of free copper to be reliable, the analyses of serum for ceruloplasmin and total copper must be accurate.

Tests of liver function should include measurements of serum bilirubin, aspartate and alanine aminotransferases, albumin, globulins, alkaline phosphatase and prothrombin time, as well as other tests that are appropriate for the individual patient. Table 15–1 shows how various indices of liver function changed in a group of patients with Wilson's disease receiving penicillamine therapy.

Measurement of the urinary output of copper is also useful in assessing the effectiveness of treatment. When treatment with penicillamine is begun, it is not unusual for a daily dose of one gram to be associated with the excretion of 3 to 5 or more milligrams of copper in a 24-hour period. Invariably, however, the amount of copper excreted diminishes as months or years of effective treatment pass, and a well-treated patient may excrete only 0.5 mg of copper, or less, in a day's urine—an amount that generally is little, if at all, increased by increasing the dose of penicillamine. If, in a patient who has been under treatment for years, the urinary output of copper is noted to be markedly elevated, compared with several preceding measurements, it suggests that the prescribed daily dose of penicillamine has not been taken regularly recently, except for the day on which the

TABLE 15–1. Effects of D-Penicillamine on Liver Function During the First Year of Therapy

	No. of Patients Treated		No. of Patients Improved
Albumin deficiency	18	Corrected	15
Elevated AST or ALT (SGOT or SGPT)	41	Decreased to normal	30
Prolonged prothrombin time	15	Improved	9
Jaundice, edema, ascites	16	Disappeared	12

patient collected the 24-hour urine. In patients with renal tubular acidosis (see Chapter 11) the urinary excretion of copper may be diminished.[5]

Unless the asymptomatic patient remains in this state, or the overtly ill one improves, it is probable that the daily dose of penicillamine is too low. It should be raised to 1.5 to 2 grams in such instances, and, more important, the physician must try to ascertain whether the patient has really been taking his penicillamine in the amount and manner prescribed. Unfortunately, by the time penicillamine treatment is instituted some patients have already suffered irreversible hepatic or brain damage and cannot respond favorably to the larger dose of penicillamine. However, in a few patients in whom this has seemed to be the case, the addition of a course of injections of BAL has had a beneficial effect.

Treatment carried out along these lines restores the majority of patients (including some who are very ill) to a state of good health. Yet, even when the physician is certain that they have adhered to the prescribed regimen, other patients may remain as ill as when first seen, or their disease may progress, rarely even fatally. A third group is characterized by significant improvement that, however, eventually ceases, leaving residual manifestations of the disorder. We do not know of any criteria by which one can predict in which of these three ways a particular symptomatic patient will respond to decoppering therapy. There is, however, abundant evidence that continual, adequate therapy maintains the *asymptomatic* patient in that state.[20]

Of the neurologic manifestations tremors, both resting and intention; awkward gait; illegibly scrawled handwriting; and scanned speech are the most likely to improve and not infrequently disappear with treatment. In contrast, dysarthria associated with dystonically immobile facial muscles that has progressed in extreme instances to mutism; and dystonic rigidity of arms, hands, legs and feet, often with contractures requiring surgical intervention, are less likely to improve, and almost never disappear. Despite studies of the nature of the dysarthrias seen,[21] speech therapy has not often proven to be of significant adjuvant value to penicillamine treatment in our patients.

The effect of treatment on the psychiatric disturbances of Wilson's disease is unpredictable, as is apparent from Chapter 9. In adolescents it is difficult to know whether the impaired memory, the inability to concentrate and the sudden deterioration of school work that may occur—manifestations that are probably partly neurologic and partly psychiatric—are direct effects of copper toxicosis or a consequence of the patient's preoccupation with his sense that his body is no longer operating correctly. It is surprising how often this triad improves with treatment.

With treatment, hepatocytic dysfunction improves remarkably and the hepatic concentration of copper tends to decrease (Table 15–2). The patient's nutritional status tends to improve dramatically, particularly if dysphagia (sometimes a total inability to swallow) responds to penicillamine. Edema and ascites generally disappear provided that the routine measures used for them, which are ineffective if used alone, are combined with adequate penicillamine treatment. Portal hypertension and, of course, splenomegaly and hypersplenic effects change little with penicillamine treatment, although we have the impression that, at least in some patients, the frequency of episodes of hematemesis from esophageal

TABLE 15–2. Clinical and Morphologic Hepatic Data on Seven Patients with Wilson's Disease

Patient	Age (in years)		Hepatic Copper (mcg/g dry weight)		Aminotransferases (AST/ALT)		Significant Morphologic Changes in Liver Biopsy Specimens During Interval of Study
	At Diagnosis	*At Follow-up*	*At Diagnosis*	*At Follow-up*	*At Diagnosis*	*At Follow-up*	
F1	15	18	821	109	52/59	39/20	Marked diminution of steatosis; persistence of mild fibrosis; normalization of apposition of mitochondrial membranes and of appearance of matrix; proliferation of endoplasmic reticulum; increase in lipofuscin
S14	9	13	1004	945	76/136	20/44	Marked diminution of steatosis; irregular improvement of mitochondrial changes, varying in magnitude from cell to cell; more glycogen nuclei and lipofuscin
S13	12	16	866	737	180/190	24/26	Marked diminution of mitochondrial abnormalities (follow-up histologic section inadequate for evaluation of changes in the steatosis, fibrosis and cellular infiltrates orginally present)

S12	15	19	1123	239	22/94	16/22	Disappearance of severe steatosis, cellular infiltrates and glycogen nuclei; marked improvement in appearance of mitochondria; persistence of lipofuscin
M10	10	15	832	453	57/88	53/48	Diminution of steatosis; disappearance of cellular infiltrates; persistence of mild fibrosis and glycogen nuclei; subsidence of initially mild mitochondrial abnormalities
HB1*	12	15	1177	1050	65/85	45/43	Diminution of severe steatosis and fibrosis; disappearance of cellular infiltrates; persistence of irregularly distributed mitochondrial abnormalities
HB2*	14	17	—	—	75/82	50/35	Persistence of cirrhosis; diminution of steatosis, cellular infiltrates and altered mitochondria.

*Patients treated at Hôpital Beaujon, Clichy, France.

From Sternlieb, I., and Feldmann, G. Gastroenterology *71*:457–461, 1976. With permission of the publisher.

varices may diminish with time. Several years ago, together with Walshe, we reported that a medical regimen is as useful for the management of the latter as is surgery.[21a] Yet in two patients, A5 and B5, both of whom had had several life-threatening hematemeses over a period of several months, splenectomy and construction of a splenorenal shunt (during which aneurysms of the splenic artery, in addition to prominent varices, were seen in A5) have so far kept A5 free of any further bleeding for seven years, and B5 for 21 years.

Perhaps the most striking evidence for the therapeutic effect of D-penicillamine on the liver is the fact that neither fulminant hepatitis with hemolysis nor hepatic decompensation has occurred in patients receiving continual therapy, whereas one or the other has developed in at least eight patients (fatally in five) who interrupted treatment for periods of nine months to three years.

There have been few investigations of the effects of long-term penicillamine treatment on morphologic changes in the liver, probably because in only a very few patients has it seemed necessary to repeat a biopsy of the liver to determine changes in the copper concentration of this organ and its histopathologic state (Table 15–2). In a study of 17 patients Mareček et al. found decreased hepatic copper concentration and improved histology after years of penicillamine treatment.[21b]

In 1975 Grand and Vawter[22] reported histopathologic findings on seven patients treated for periods ranging from two to seven years. In only two of the four patients in whom pretreatment biopsies had been performed was there considerable reduction in portal fibrosis; in three, therapy had greatly lessened portal inflammation and necrosis; but in none had normal histology been restored. In six of seven young patients in Table 15–2, the prominent steatosis, cellular infiltrates and mitochondrial abnormalities observed at the time of diagnosis had largely subsided after three to four years of treatment, although fibrosis persisted.[23] Indeed, in contrast to one report of a child in whom disappearance of fibrosis was observed in serial biopsy samples of the liver, [24] we have never seen convincing evidence in any of our patients of a significant reduction in the amount of excess collagen.

Almost invariably girls who have never menstruated or who have had irregular or abnormal periods as a consequence of Wilson's disease establish normal cycles with effective penicillamine treatment. Puberty, occasionally delayed in the untreated boy or girl, progresses normally with specific therapy. The repeated miscarriages seen in untreated Wilson's disease, probably due to the abnormally high concentration of copper ions in endometrial secretions,[25] are not seen in treated patients, who seem normal in their ability to conceive and deliver healthy babies. It is more likely that women with adequately treated Wilson's disease will deliver normal infants without exacerbation of their disease if they continue to receive penicillamine throughout pregnancy.[26–28] (See Chapter 16.)

What is the outlook for patients with Wilson's disease since the U.S. Food and Drug Administration approved D-penicillamine as safe and effective for this illness in 1963? Of 33 patients reported in 1964,[2] 19 are still alive. Of these, five were then, and still continue to be, asymptomatic;

seven have become so on treatment; and all 12 live normally in all respects. Among the other patients, three have residual neurologic disability, and three still exhibit psychiatric abnormalities. The remaining patient, S4, remained asymptomatic while on treatment from the age of 6 to 16, and then discontinued penicillamine voluntarily. Four years later, despite several hospitalizations, courses of BAL and exhortations that he resume taking penicillamine regularly, he is almost totally neurologically incapacitated.

Of the 14 patients who are dead, three (A2, M1 and R9) succumbed to hepatic insufficiency following discontinuance of penicillamine treatment. Three (B6, G6 and M4), in whom it is uncertain whether penicillamine was being taken in adequate dosage, died of unknown causes. Two patients (D6 and P6) died of hepatic insufficiency while taking penicillamine. In P6 overt liver dysfunction developed within weeks following a pregnancy during which she took no penicillamine. Despite continued penicillamine therapy, two patients (M2 and T3) exsanguinated from esophageal varices; two (S16 and T7) died of postoperative infection; one (E4), of ovarian carcinoma; and one (P4), of an unknown cause while receiving penicillamine in a mental hospital.

Although they are of no permanent, significant clinical benefit if their use is not accompanied by the administration of an adequate dosage of penicillamine or triethylene tetramine (Trien), several drugs and one procedure have been used as adjuvants to decoppering therapy.

L-Dopa was first used in 1970, by Barbeau and Friesen,[29] in a 15-year-old girl with Wilson's disease whose neurologic manifestations deteriorated over 15 months while she was receiving two grams of penicillamine daily. (The development of dermatopathy characteristic of this dose afforded evidence that she was, in fact, taking the penicillamine.) The addition of one gram of L-dopa daily and 200 mg of a decarboxylase inhibitor resulted in marked functional improvement within two months. Unfortunately, longer follow-up has not been reported. The addition of L-dopa for seven months to regimens based on either penicillamine or Trien in a 14-year-old boy,[30] and a 12-year-old girl[31] also proved beneficial. Substitution, in the latter case, of a placebo for the L-dopa was followed by relapse of neurologic symptoms. But failure of L-dopa to improve such symptoms was reported in the case of a 36-year-old woman receiving penicillamine.[32]

In a young woman, P7, whose severe dysarthria, dystonic rigidity, and contractures had improved very little after four years of adequate treatment with penicillamine, a trial of L-dopa was without effect. In another young patient of ours, G2, with severe rigidity and dysarthria persisting after a year of penicillamine treatment, the addition of L-dopa to, and the removal of pyridoxine from, her regimen was followed by gradual amelioration in speech and rigidity. The improvement continued even after the L-dopa was withdrawn. Other antiparkinsonian drugs have not afforded symptomatic relief from rigidity or, indeed, from tremors.

The administration of L-dopa must not be accompanied by pyridoxine because of its antagonism to L-dopa's activity. However, since the evidence for the need for pyridoxine in patients receiving penicillamine comes solely from animal experiments, and since we have never observed any adverse effect in those patients who have omitted taking pyridoxine for months, we believe that there is little risk in discontinuing pyridoxine if a patient taking penicillamine is clearly benefited by L-dopa.

Phenobarbital, diphenyl hydantoin or both have been successful in controlling grand mal seizures in three of our patients, A4, C3, and E2, in the first two of whom elimination of these drugs has not been followed by any further episodes.

SIDE EFFECTS OF PENICILLAMINE AND THEIR MANAGEMENT

Early side effects, apparently allergic, are manifested by fever, rash, lymphadenopathy, leukopenia, thrombocytopenia or some combination of these. Reactions of this sort are generally seen between the end of the first and third weeks following the institution of therapy, and they occur in about 20 per cent of patients with Wilson's disease.[2]

Fever, which we have seen reach 41°C, almost always accompanies a *rash*, which may be diffusely erythematous, macular, slightly papular and/or pruritic. Occasionally mucosae are involved.

Lymphadenopathy, sometimes generalized, is more commonly localized to the nodes of the neck.

Granulocytopenia, agranulocytosis and *thrombocytopenia* are much more unusual, and more serious, early reactions.[2, 8, 33, 34] Since leukopenia, granulocytopenia or thrombocytopenia may be a consequence of the hypersplenism that often is part of Wilson's disease, pretreatment white blood cell, differential and platelet counts (estimates of the last from a smear are not sufficiently accurate) must be obtained.

In our experience and that of other investigators it has always been possible to desensitize patients with early fever and rash, making possible the eventual institution of continual penicillamine administration[2, 34–37] When either appears, the drug should be stopped immediately and no more given until the reactions have completely subsided. In some patients it is then sufficient to reinstitute penicillamine administration in markedly reduced dosages of about 10 to 25 mg daily, with a gradual increase over a month or more to full 1 g/day dosage, without recurrence of sensitivity.

> **Eleven days after penicillamine treatment was instituted in D1, a 12-year-old asymptomatic girl, an urticarial eruption began on her neck, spread down to involve her thighs, and soon became macular and pruritic. There was no fever. Penicillamine was discontinued for three days and, the rash having disappeared, was reinstituted at 10 mg daily and increased gradually. Within a month a dose of one gram daily had been achieved with no further reaction.**

Although management of this sort was our usual practice more than 10 years ago, we have since found it preferable to administer a corticosteroid—about 20 to 30 mg of prednisone or its equivalent—beginning two or three days before the reinstitution of penicillamine. Then the latter is given at a dosage of 0.25 g daily for about three to five days, and full dosage can be attained gradually over about two weeks. If no reaction recurs, the steroid may be tapered to zero a week or two later. Fever, rash or both may recur even in the presence of steroid, in which case penicillamine should be discontinued a second time, with maintenance of the steroid. Again, on subsidence of the reaction, penicillamine is reinstituted in somewhat more gradually increasing dosages from an initial 0.125 g (since capsules of this size are available) daily.

Within two weeks after the institution of penicillamine therapy in A5, a boy of 11, fever to 38.5°C led to its discontinuation. Three days later, when he was afebrile, the drug was readministered in a one-gram daily dosage; within three days a fine maculopapular eruption appeared on his trunk and his temperature rose to 38°C. Again penicillamine was withdrawn for four days and then given in a dose of one gram, together with 20 mg of prednisone, daily. For three weeks no reaction was noted, and the prednisone was tapered. When the daily dose of the latter reached 7.5 mg, a macular eruption appeared on his calves and thighs and his temperature spiked to 40.2°C. Prednisone was increased to 15 mg daily, and penicillamine was withdrawn for three days and then reinstituted at one gram daily. Ten days later, temperature rose sharply to 41.5°C, accompanied by a nonproductive cough. Prednisone was raised to 20 mg daily, and penicillamine discontinued. Over the next month, prednisone was continued at the same dosage and penicillamine reintroduced at 0.25 g daily. With no further reaction, a month later, when he was receiving one gram penicillamine daily, the prednisone was gradually reduced to zero. No further reaction to penicillamine has occurred in the ensuing 22 years.

Evidence of significant marrow depression requires immediate withdrawal of penicillamine. Steroids are of no value in the treatment of penicillamine-induced granulocytopenia, although they may be of help if thrombocytopenia develops. When counts have returned to their pretreatment values, very cautious and gradual reinstitution of penicillamine may be attempted, beginning with no more than 0.01 g daily for at least a week. In one patient, M4, leukopenia and thrombocytopenia developed as reactions to penicillamine; both eventually were reversed within 2½ months after penicillamine treatment, accompanied by steroids, was begun.

Attempts at desensitization to hematologic reactions of these sorts are rarely, if ever, undertaken in patients receiving penicillamine for the treatment of rheumatoid arthritis. With Wilson's disease, however, we are concerned with a disorder that is progressive and fatal. Consequently, we have risked reinstitution of penicillamine in several patients with such serious reactions, successfully in about half of them, and with no permanent ill effects in any.

Late reactions to penicillamine are generally seen after the first year of continual therapy. The longer a patient has been receiving a daily dose of penicillamine of one gram or less, the less likely is the occurrence of serious reactions. Yet even fatal toxicity of the drug can occur years after treatment has successfully controlled the patient's Wilson's disease, as in patient G1, who died of penicillamine-induced Goodpasture's syndrome (Figs. 15–1 and 15–2). Patients must remain under a physician's continued and regular observation for life. The following late reactions to penicillamine have been observed.

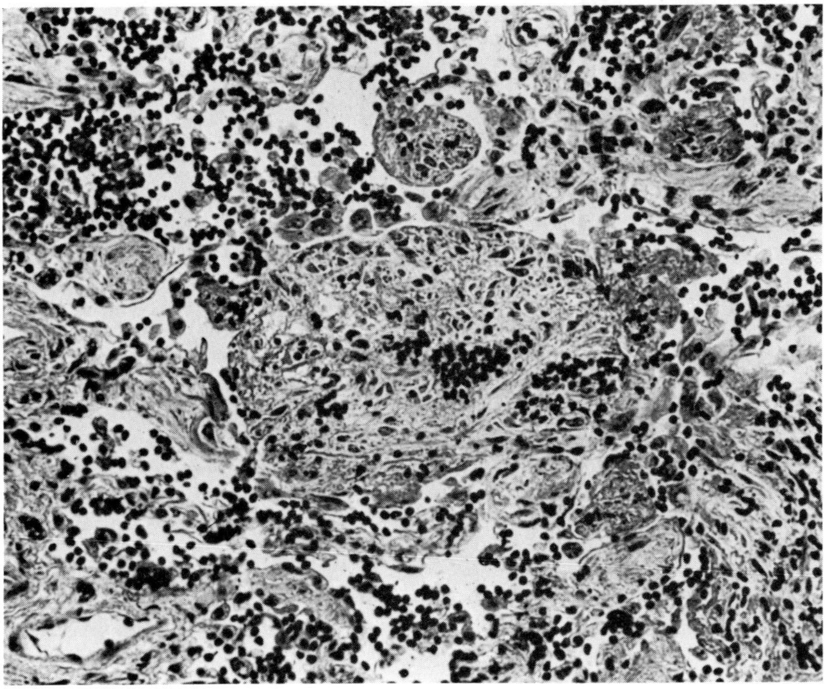

Figure 15–1. Thickening of alveolar septal walls and hemorrhage in the lungs of patient G1, who succumbed to Goodpasture's syndrome. Autopsy specimen. Hematoxylin-eosin. × 400.

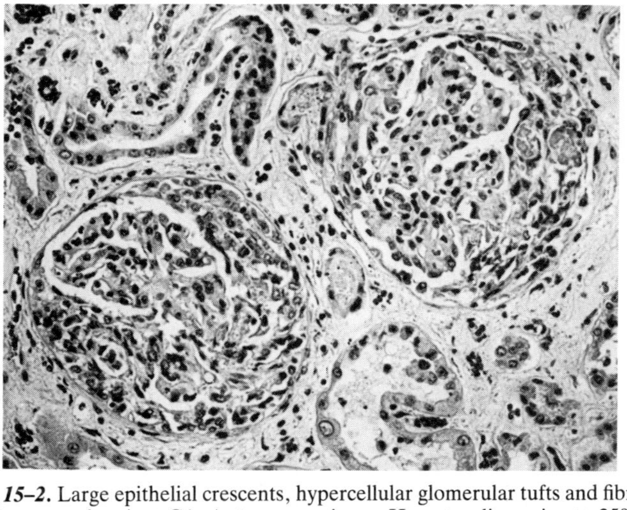

Figure 15–2. Large epithelial crescents, hypercellular glomerular tufts and fibrin deposits in the renal cortex of patient G1. Autopsy specimen. Hematoxylin-eosin. × 250.

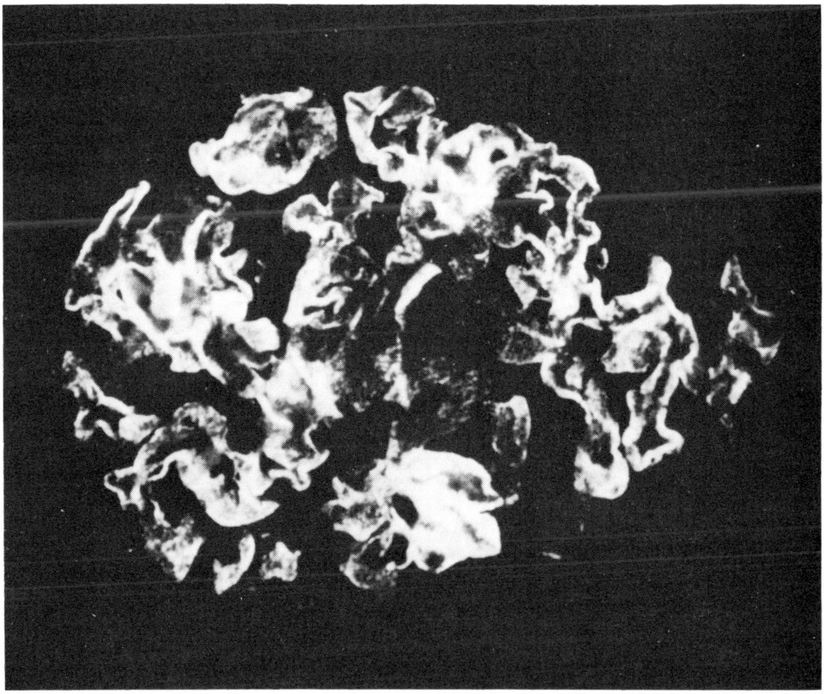

Figure 15–3. Granular pattern of antibody to human IgG distributed along the glomerular basement membrane. Renal biopsy specimen. Patient Y1 with nephrotic syndrome. × 1000. (Courtesy Dr. B. Bennett.)

1. *Nephrotoxicity*. Although about 20 per cent of patients receiving penicillamine for rheumatoid arthritis may manifest severe proteinuria or the nephrotic syndrome,[38] such penicillamine-induced immune complex nephropathy (Figs. 15–3 and 15–4) has occurred in fewer than 5 per cent of patients with Wilson's disease, in our experience, and in 10 per cent in that of Lössner et al.[39–43] Mild and stable proteinuria of less than about 0.5 g daily is compatible with the continuation of penicillamine therapy in Wilson's disease. With proteinuria over one gram daily, the drug should be reduced in dosage, and it should be discontinued if significant proteinuria persists. Cautious and gradual reinstitution of penicillamine (with simultaneous administration of corticosteroids in some instances) may not provoke a recurrence of proteinuria. But in a few patients, persistently elevated proteinuria or a full-blown nephrotic syndrome (despite corticosteroids) has required changing the patient's medication to Trien.[9, 39, 44, 45]

2. *Systemic lupus erythematosus*. Usually preceded by proteinuria and hematuria, the form of lupus seen in penicillamine-treated Wilson's disease patients is often accompanied by arthralgias and is distinguishable from immune complex nephropathy.[46–48] The diagnosis of lupus generally requires the demonstration of both fluorescent nuclear antibody, and LE cells, but the latter are sometimes absent even when the diagnosis seems rather certain. The administration of corticosteroids in low dosage, equivalent to 5 to 10 mg of prednisone daily and indefinitely, has been somewhat

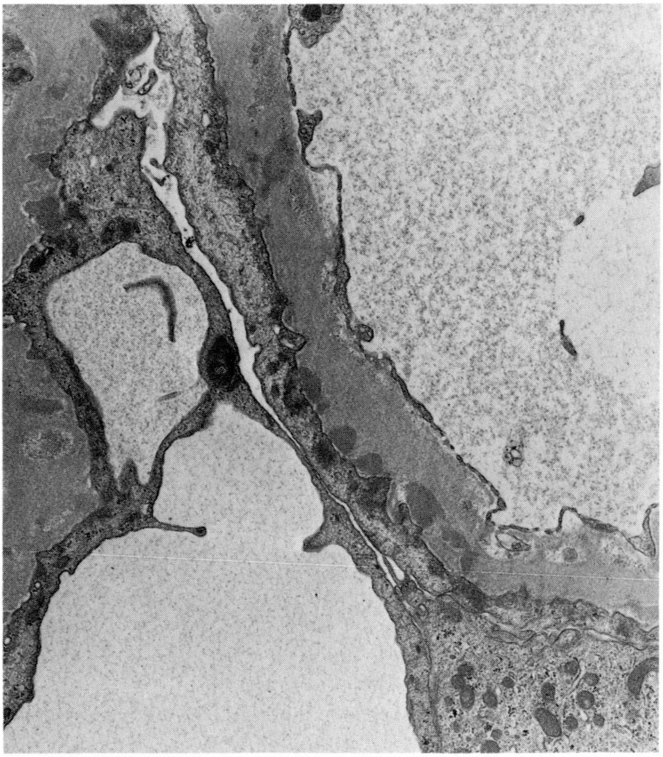

Figure 15–4. Portion of glomerular capillary loop showing epimembranous and intramembranous electron-dense deposits and effacement of the foot processes. Renal biopsy specimen. Patient Y1. Electron micrograph. × 27,000. (Courtesy Dr. R. Janis.)

more effective in keeping lupus under control than in controlling immune complex nephropathy, although the dosage of penicillamine may have to be somewhat less than optimal, at 0.5 g daily. If such a regimen is not adequate for control of both the lupus and the Wilson's disease, penicillamine must be replaced by Trien.

3. *Thrombocytopenia*. Apparently induced by penicillamine, thrombocytopenia has been seen in several patients with Wilson's disease.[2, 27, 33] In evaluating platelet counts made during treatment it must be borne in mind, as already mentioned, that patients with Wilson's disease who suffer from hypersplenism may exhibit pre–penicillamine-treatment platelet counts of less than 100,000/cu mm.[27, 49] We have been able to maintain a number of patients on successful penicillamine therapy, despite platelet counts of about 50,000/cu mm, with no evidence of abnormal bleeding or bruising. If platelet counts drop as low as about 25,000, however, penicillamine may have to be discontinued. In these patients its reinstitution has invariably been accompanied by recurrence of dangerous thrombocytopenia despite reduction in the dose of penicillamine, or of simultaneous corticosteroid therapy. In such instances, as with severe renal disease, Trien will have to be used. A fatal case of thrombohemolytic thrombocytopenic purpura (Moschcowitz's syndrome) due to penicillamine has been reported.[50]

4. *Agranulocytosis*. We have not seen agranulocytosis as a *late* reaction to penicillamine, although we perform white blood cell counts each time a patient is seen. An instance of red cell aplasia occurring after 14 years of treatment has been reported by Gollan et al.[51]

5. *Optic axial neuritis*. This disorder, with severe visual disturbance, has occurred in three patients who received D,L-penicillamine[52–54] but has not been reported in patients receiving D-penicillamine, the only form of the drug currently marketed.

6. *Goodpasture's syndrome*. In three patients with Wilson's disease who had at some time received penicillamine therapy in excess of one gram daily, pulmonary and renal hemorrhages heralded the onset of fatal Goodpasture's syndrome.[55] Urine should be examined for blood at least every six months, and patients should be alerted to look for and report immediately hemoptysis or the appearance of blood in the urine. Particularly in children, however, microscopic hematuria may be a feature of untreated Wilson's disease; if it does not progress, it is not a contraindication to continuing the regimen (see Chapter 11).

7. *Skin reactions*. The commonest late reactions of penicillamine therapy in Wilson's disease are seen in the skin.

a. Two or more grams of penicillamine, given daily for more than several months, generally cause what has been termed *penicillamine dermatopathy*.[2, 56–58] This dosage of penicillamine interferes with cross-

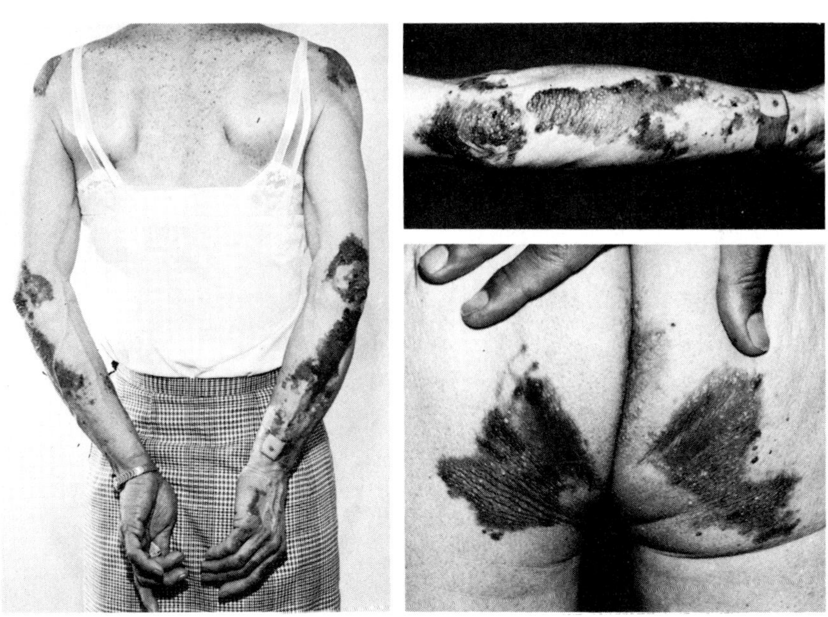

Figure 15–5. Characteristic lesions of penicillamine dermatopathy on the shoulders, elbows, extensor surfaces of the forearms and buttocks of patient E4. This patient received approximately 4 g/day of D-penicillamine for the three years preceding these pictures. Similar lesions were present on the knees, shins and dorsa of both feet. The large blotchy, flat areas were purplish red. White papules are seen within the purpuric areas. (With the permission of The Journal of Rheumatology *8*[Suppl. 7]:149–154, 1981, and The Journal of the American Medical Association, Sept. 7, 1964, *189*:748–754. Copyright 1964, American Medical Association.)

linking of collagen and elastin[59] and results in weakening of subcutaneous tissue, so that slight trauma—the pressure of a brassiere strap, or of a hard chair on the buttocks—may cause bleeding into subcutaneous tissues (Fig. 15–5). On healing, areas of brown skin and white papules ranging in size from one to several millimeters in diameter usually remain. Histologic examination of these lesions demonstrates cords of degenerative stroma, focal granulomatous inflammation, proliferation of small capillaries and keratin-filled cysts (Fig. 15–6). This dermatopathy, and animal experiments in which penicillamine has been found to impair wound healing[60] have led us to recommend reduction of penicillamine to 0.25 to 0.5 g daily for three to six weeks following and, if possible, preceding major surgery.

After years of treatment, penicillamine can produce a more subtle effect on the skin—progeric wrinkling, particularly of the neck, face and axillary folds. The appearance of women so distressingly affected[61] may be that of someone years older. This rarely occurs, however, unless the daily dose of penicillamine exceeds one gram, and since current practice is to prescribe no more than that for most patients, both penicillamine-induced dermatopathy and wrinkling (Fig. 15–7) are no longer often seen.

b. *Elastosis perforans serpiginosa (EPS)*, a disorder generally thought to be idiopathic, has been seen in patients with Wilson's disease after years of penicillamine therapy.[56, 62–64] Unlike the dermatopathy just described, EPS does not seem to be dose related, and though it occurs in female patients, it seems to be commoner in males. The lesions are raised, arcuate, but not completely circular (Fig. 15–8). They appear singly or in groups, on the neck and axillae most frequently, but they have also been noted on the arms, the trunk, the chin, the penis and in the antecubital fossae (Fig. 15–9). Generally symptomless (except for the lesions' significant cosmetic effects), EPS occasionally causes mild itching or burning. Biopsy samples of the lesions show that elastin has herniated up through the dermis, distorting the dermal and epidermal architecture. No treatment has proven effective, though abrasive removal or keratinolytic agents may be of marginal value. Reduction of dosage has not seemed to affect existing lesions, but in at least two patients, G3 and M6, the lesions, after persisting for years, have almost completely disappeared despite continued penicillamine therapy in unchanged dosage. Cryotherapy with liquid nitrogen has been reported to result in disappearance of EPS lesions without scarring in one patient.[64a]

c. *Pemphigus*, or pemphigoid lesions, have been reported in several patients receiving penicillamine (see Color Plate 2, Figure 5; and Fig. 15–10).[65, 66]

d. *Lichen planus*, apparently related to penicillamine therapy, has been seen in Wilson's disease.[56, 67]

e. Painful *aphthous stomatitis,* severe enough to interfere seriously with eating, has been attributed to penicillamine in a few patients with Wilson's disease.[67, 68]

8. *Anaphylaxis*. In a patient of ours, C1, a physician treated successfully for more than 20 years with penicillamine, a two-week interruption of the drug was followed by severe, obstructive laryngeal edema within minutes of swallowing the first capsule of penicillamine. Since then, following any interruption in its daily administration, we observe and

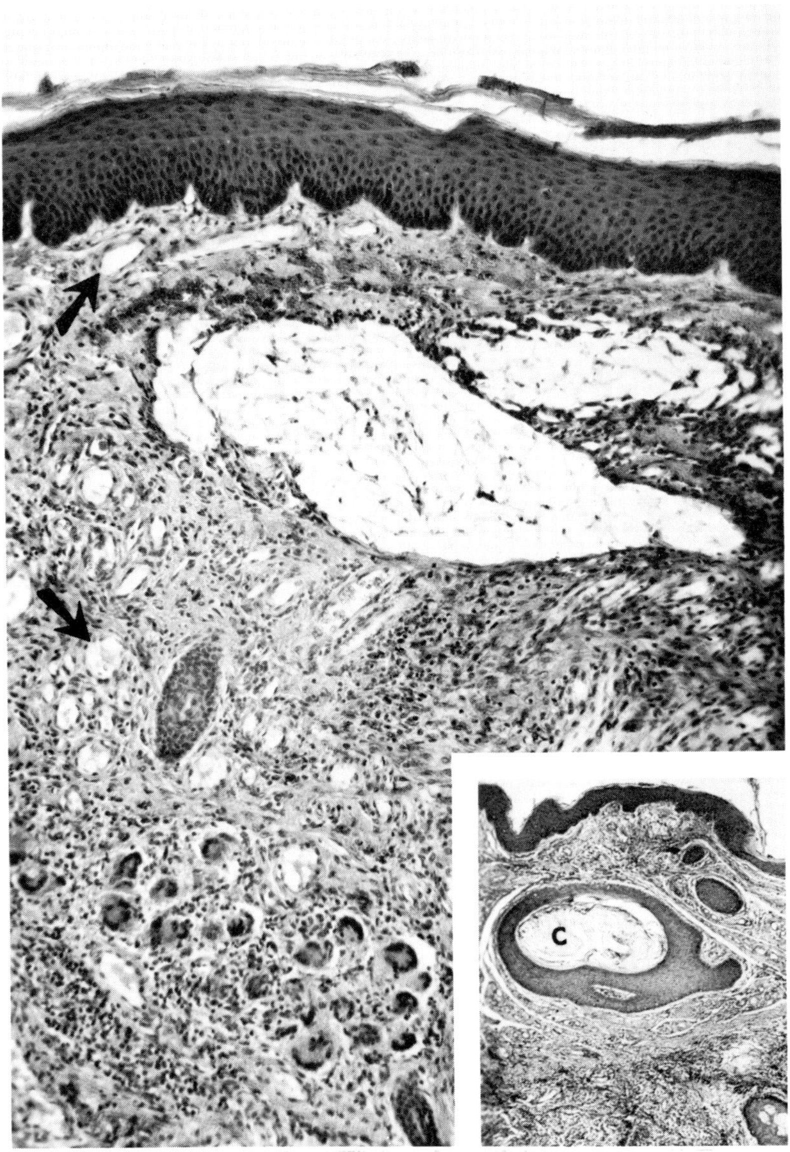

Figure 15–6. Proliferation of small capillaries *(arrow)* surrounding cords of degenerative stroma with focal inflammation in the perianal skin from patient E4. *Inset:* A small keratin-filled cyst *(c)* lined by squamous cells. Skin biopsy. Hematoxylin-eosin. × 115. *Inset:* × 40. (With the permission of The Journal of Rheumatology *8*[Suppl. 7]:149–154, 1981, and The Journal of the American Medical Association, Sept. 7, 1964, *189*:748–754. Copyright 1964, American Medical Association.)

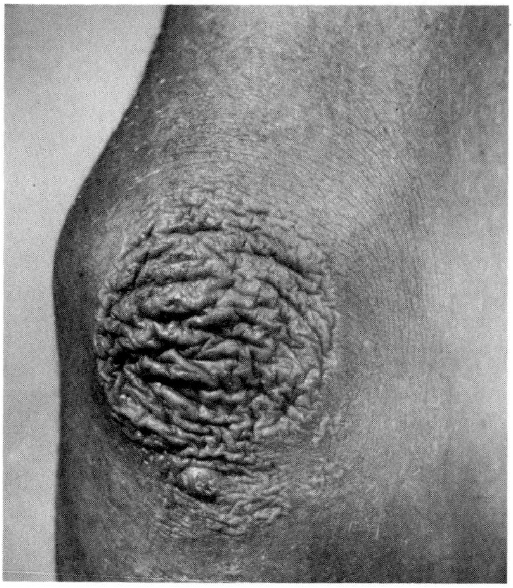

Figure 15–7. Excessive wrinkling and thinning of skin at site of previous penicillamine dermatopathy on elbow of patient M6 at 18 years of age. (With the permission of The Journal of Rheumatology *8*[Suppl. 7]:149–154, 1981.)

caution patients about the possibility of sensitivity to penicillamine just as though it were being first administered. Patients should be warned *never* to stop the drug, either intentionally or inadvertently, and to reduce the dosage to 0.25 g daily if a low supply of medication cannot be replenished in time to permit continuing full dosage.

9. *Myasthenia gravis*. Reported in two patients with Wilson's disease, myasthenia gravis has been associated with IgG and C3 deposition within a hyperplastic thymus. In one, with elevated levels of antibody to acetylcholine receptor in the gland,[69] mild anticholinesterase therapy controlled the myasthenia despite continued penicillamine treatment. In the other patient the myasthenia disappeared and reappeared when penicillamine was discontinued and readministered.[70]

10. *Loss of taste*. A not infrequent symptom in patients receiving penicillamine for rheumatoid arthritis, loss of taste is much rarer in patients with Wilson's disease. Although when first reported[71] this phenomenon was thought to be associated with deficiency of copper, this proved difficult to reconcile with the fact that taste generally returned even if copper was not added to the diet and treatment with penicillamine was not interrupted. Later speculation that zinc deficiency might be a cause of this symptom[72] has also remained unconfirmed.

11. *Depression of IgA levels in serum.* There have been reports of a marked depression in the serum concentration of IgA in isolated penicillamine-treated patients with Wilson's disease in Belgium,[73] Sweden,[74, 75] Great Britain,[51] and France,[76] and in six of 40 patients investigated by Strickland and Leu in Taiwan.[77] Czlonkowska found significantly lower levels of IgA, IgG, and IgM immunoglobulins, as well as of two antibodies to bacterial antigens, in eight patients with Wilson's disease treated for

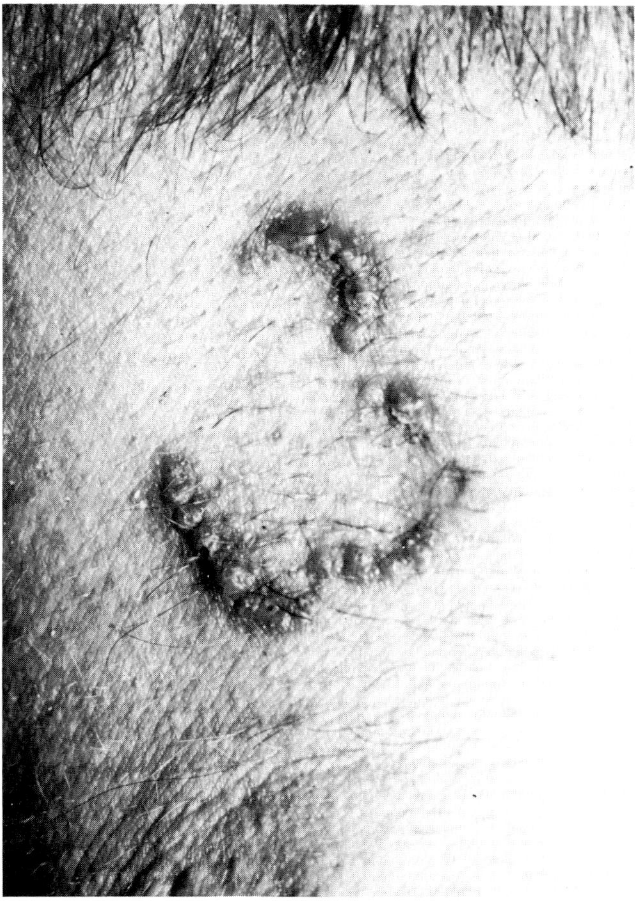

Figure 15–8. Raised, delled papules coalesced to form a large arcuate lesion, characteristic of elastosis perforans serpiginosa, on the back of the neck of patient B3 after 12 years of treatment with D-penicillamine. (With the permission of the Archives of Dermatology, Nov. 1973, *108*:713–715. Copyright 1973, American Medical Association.)

istration will often cause massive hematomata and there is no evidence of its value.

2. Equally critically ill is the patient who typically presents with dystonic rigidity of his entire body, usually in the fetal position; with inability to walk, talk, swallow or close his mouth; with fingers, wrists, and elbows generally immovably fixed in flexion; and with uselessly rigid legs and equinovarus feet. Like the patient whose liver disease is life-endangering, but unlike the violently tremulous patient who may be just as incapacitated but who is likely to respond favorably to therapy, the patient with such severe dystonia is usually terminally ill. Rarely, with intensive therapy and nursing care,[80c] a patient of this sort will survive and recover fully.

After a regimen has been established to provide nutrition for what is likely to be a period of months, therapy should consist of 2.0 g of penicillamine daily in four divided doses administered, if necessary, by nasogastric tube, and 3.0 ml of BAL in one or two doses administered intramuscularly three to five times a week.

This regimen should be continued for at least a month (two months, if the BAL does not cause intolerable intramuscular bleeding or abscesses) before the administration of BAL is interrupted. If improvement has been achieved, BAL should be reinstituted after a week or two of respite.

The site of administration of BAL should alternate daily between the right and left buttocks. Each injection should be one to two inches lower than that of the prior injection in that buttock, avoiding the sciatic nerve. With about five sites available in each buttock it is often possible to return to the original injection site in two weeks and continue the course. A diagram of dates and sites of injections, kept at the patient's bedside or in the chart, is useful.

The rationale of adding BAL to penicillamine therapy in such extremely ill patients stems from the fact that it, in contrast to penicillamine, is electrically uncharged and is probably able to cross vascular and cellular membranes more readily than penicillamine, with its charged carboxyl and amino groups. BAL may, therefore, accelerate the removal of copper from within brain tissue.[81, 82]

Perhaps for the same reason BAL is occasionally of significant value in treating neurologically affected patients who, though not incapacitated, have not responded with great clinical improvement to penicillamine. It can frequently be administered to such patients in the physician's office or at home by a trained nurse or physician's assistant.

TREATMENT OF THE PSYCHIATRICALLY DISTURBED PATIENT

In contrast to the hepatic and neurologic manifestations of Wilson's disease, the psychiatric disturbances (see Chapter 9) not only result from the toxic effects of copper on the integrative centers of the brain but also constitute reactions to the catastrophic physical effects of the illness. Consequently, unless the emotional disturbances are minimal, penicillamine alone will not restore the patient to normal occupational or family roles. Psychotherapy and appropriate psychotropic medications must be administered *pari passu* with decoppering therapy. For severely disturbed patients, some of whom are suicidal, clinical management must be undertaken cooperatively by the physician (treating the copper toxicosis) and a psychiatrist, psychologist, or psychiatric social worker.

The therapeutic results of such combined decoppering and psychologic therapy are often—but, unfortunately, not always—gratifying. In some of these patients, lifelong supportive psychotherapy and occasional, sometimes protracted, inpatient psychiatric care are necessary.

Psychologic treatment of these patients should be the same as would be appropriate if the disturbance manifested were present in a patient without Wilson's disease. Surprisingly, some psychiatrists and psychologists, believing that the patient with Wilson's disease has a purely "organic" brain disturbance and should be treated only pharmacologically, may be reluctant to provide psychotherapy. From our experience we have no doubt that psychotherapy and judiciously used medications (though not electric shock or insulin coma) can be almost as important to the patient's well-being as penicillamine.

TREATMENT OF THE ASYMPTOMATIC PATIENT

Since untreated Wilson's disease has been known for almost 75 years to be uniformly progressive and fatal it must be obvious that the asymptomatic patient with a confirmed diagnosis of Wilson's disease must be treated for his entire life as intensively as is necessary to keep him free of any overt manifestation of the illness.[83–98] Experience of more than 20 years in more than a hundred patients has confirmed that failure to do so inevitably leads to signs and symptoms that may be irreversible, or to death.[20] Most of these patients take penicillamine regularly and remain asymptomatic indefinitely. But in several of our patients, years of good health have been followed by a more or less gradual deterioration and the appearance of classic signs and symptoms of Wilson's disease. These are patients who have come to believe that their years of normality have not been the result of the penicillamine they have taken, and who have consequently become lax in their adherence to their regimen or have even stopped taking any penicillamine. In most cases, the eventual appearance of tremors, drooling, hemolytic anemia, hepatitis or some other symptom or sign convinces the patient of his misconception, and the reinstitution of penicillamine is followed by a return to the asymptomatic state. In other patients, however, because the pathologic effects that have developed during interruption of treatment are irreversible or because the patient does not begin, or continue, taking penicillamine, illness persists, worsens or ends fatally.

TREATMENT OF THE PATIENT INTOLERANT TO PENICILLAMINE

1. *BAL.* This is available as a 10 per cent suspension in peanut oil, and must be administered intramuscularly. It is not a practical alternative to penicillamine for the lifelong treatment necessary for Wilson's disease,

but it has brought a number of severely ill patients with Wilson's disease back to a state of good health and has resulted in significant improvement in others.[81, 82, 99] Generally, for the reasons given above, its use must be in courses of several weeks with periods of interruption. It is available commercially in the United States, though not specifically approved by the Food and Drug Administration for Wilson's disease.

2. *Triethylene tetramine dihydrochloride (Trien, Trientine, TETA).* In 1968 Walshe introduced this practical alternative to penicillamine.[9, 44, 100] The drug is given orally in doses of about 1 to 1.5 grams daily. Although in our limited experience Trien does not usually produce the degree of cupriuresis that penicillamine does, its continued use is undoubtedly therapeutically effective. It has been designated by the U.S. Food and Drug Administration as an "orphan drug" for the treatment of penicillamine-intolerant patients with Wilson's disease.[100a]

Walshe has used Trien in 20 patients who had developed a systemic immunologic reaction to penicillamine; toxicity manifest in bone marrow, kidneys, joints, skin or buccal mucosa; or more than one of these effects. Of those in whom long-term follow-up studies were made, eight had received no significant prior treatment with penicillamine before Trien therapy was instituted, at which time five were neurologically affected; one had had acute hepatitis with hemolysis; and two were asymptomatic. From 14 months to 10 years later all but one, in whom there was residual dysarthria, were free of symptoms. Kayser-Fleischer rings had disappeared in one and diminished in the others.[100]

Of the other 12 patients, eight were asymptomatic and four exhibited residual neurologic signs at the time Trien replaced penicillamine therapy. On Trien, the eight have remained asymptomatic; the four have improved neurologically.[100]

These patients received 1.2 to 2.4 g of Trien daily. One patient took 30 grams at one time, in a suicidal attempt, with no apparent ill effects and had two subsequent successful pregnancies while still receiving Trien. Three other patients on the drug have also delivered four normal infants. Lupus nephritis developed in two patients, in only one of whom had it also been noted while he was taking penicillamine. Serum iron concentrations fell an average of 40 per cent after 40 months of Trien therapy (a phenomenon not seen with penicillamine), but rose promptly when iron was administered at bedtime some hours after the last dose of the drug.[101]

We have treated ten patients, all irreversibly intolerant to penicillamine, with Trien for about 37 patient-years and have confirmed its safety—we have observed no toxic reactions—and efficacy in maintaining the asymptomatic state or in markedly improving the symptoms and signs of Wilson's disease. Fading of Kayser-Fleischer rings has occurred in two patients, K4 and T8, while receiving Trien.

Others have reported successful treatment of single patients with Trien.[44, 45, 51, 102]

No metabolic studies of Trien have been published, but Walshe's observations indicate that copper mobilized by Trien is principally excreted in the urine.[101]

Because penicillamine is so effective, readily available and relatively cheap, we make strenuous efforts to overcome any reactions to it before considering the use of Trien. We have found it necessary to use the latter in only the approximately 2 per cent of our patients in whom recurrent nephrotic syndrome, persistent proteinuria of a gram or more daily, lupus, pemphigus or thrombocytopenia have developed. We have also substituted Trien for penicillamine in an adolescent girl, O2, in whom facial elastosis perforans serpiginosa was a severe cosmetic problem, although Walshe reported no regression of this skin lesion in one similarly managed patient, and no improvement has been seen in the EPS lesions of our patient O2—indeed new lesions have appeared—after two years on Trien.[100]

OTHER MODES OF THERAPY

Pharmacologic Therapy

1. *Zinc.* Because zinc has been reported to inhibit absorption of copper, two patients were given 200 mg of zinc sulfate daily. After 14 years, tremors (and Kayser-Fleischer rings) had disappeared, and dysarthria and rigidity had improved sufficiently to permit one of these patients to return to factory work.[103] Encouraging results over a brief period of therapy were observed in a third patient.[104] Brewer et al. have reported that the daily administration of 150 mg of elemental zinc, given as the acetate, induces negative copper balance in patients with Wilson's disease.[104a] Walshe treated a patient intolerant to penicillamine and Trien with 150 mg elemental zinc daily, given as the sulfate, for a year, at the end of which her clinical condition was unchanged; hepatic copper concentration had risen from 360 to 700 mcg/g dry liver, with more severe fatty change and fibrosis in the post-zinc biopsy sample; her SGOT/SGPT had risen from 21/51 to 39/88; and her urinary copper excretion had remained unchanged.[104b]

2. *Diethyldithiocarbamate (DTC).* Sunderman administered this compound, which combines with copper in vitro, to one patient and found increased fecal excretion of copper.[105] Hsia et al. could not confirm this in three patients.[106] In two severely ill women, DTC caused somnolence and EEG changes and did not affect urinary copper excretion.[107] Boudin and Pépin observed neurologic improvement in one patient, intolerant of penicillamine, after a year of treatment with DTC, but she succumbed to her liver disease.[108]

3. *Sodium 2,3-dimercaptopropane-1-sulfonate (Unithiol; DMPS).* This compound, a charged derivative of BAL that can be given intravenously, has been reported by Konovalov et al. to benefit the tremulous, but not the dystonic, patient.[109, 110]

4. *Sodium borate decahydrate; borax.* Oral administration of up to 1.5 g daily for about a month has resulted in increased cupriuresis and clinical improvement in four patients.[111]

Physical Therapy

1. In seven patients with Wilson's disease Sunderman et al.[112] measured the total copper content of sweat collected during a sauna bath and found that the average control value of 18 micrograms was raised to 106

when the patients were also given penicillamine. These investigators seriously suggested that inducing sweating be considered as an adjunct to the usual regimen.

2. Speech therapy can sometimes be of value in retraining the severely dysarthric patient, provided that decoppering therapy can improve the underlying neurologic disturbance. Similarly, physical therapy can help retrain the patient to write, eat, walk and regain working skills, again provided that the neurologic disturbances, and disabling contractures can be improved.

Surgical Therapy

1. *Stereotactic surgery.* Destruction of the pallidum or thalamus in more than 25 patients resulted in little, if any, improvement in either severe tremors or rigidity.[113–116] In two patients, direct electrical stimulation of the mesencephalic area has been reported to control tremors.[117]

2. *Shunts.* Because of bleeding esophageal varices, splenectomy and construction of a splenorenal shunt were performed in nine patients, and portacaval shunts were made in eight others. In 1970, with Walshe, we reported that only one patient from each of these two groups did well postoperatively; most deteriorated neurologically.[21a] Three other patients (A5, L6 and O3) have had splenectomies (with resection of a splenic arterial aneurysm in A5) and splenorenal shunts constructed. A5 and O3 have done well; L6 succumbed 16 years after his initial bleeding episode, soon after operative transection of his esophageal varices. Despite the rather high incidence of esophageal varices in patients with Wilson's disease, surgical intervention is indicated, we believe, only in the unusual patient with repeated and life-threatening episodes of bleeding.

A peritoneovenous shunt relieved ascites in a 15-year-old boy.[118]

3. *Splenectomy.* This procedure, for hypersplenism, is hardly ever, if ever, indicated in Wilson's disease.

4. *Orthotopic liver transplants.* Such transplants have been performed in two patients with Wilson's disease who were well one and eleven years postoperatively.[79, 119] Another patient so treated (and referred to in Chapter 14) was subsequently shown to have had non-Wilsonian liver disease associated with excess hepatic copper.[120]

A transplant may be indicated in three types of patients with Wilson's disease:[120a]

(a) Patients presenting with a clinical picture of fulminant hepatitis;

(b) Young cirrhotic patients with laboratory findings of severe hepatic decompensation (profound hypoalbuminemia, uncorrectable hypoprothrombinemia, progressive hyperbilirubinemia and anemia) who have failed to improve after 2 to 3 months of adequate chelation with D-penicillamine and nonspecific therapy for water retention, electrolyte balance and encephalopathy; and

(c) Effectively treated patients in whom severe, progressive hepatic insufficiency and hemolysis, clinically similar to fulminant hepatitis, develops acutely following their discontinuance of penicillamine.

5. *Tendon and muscle releasing procedures.* Such procedures have been carried out in three of our patients with crippling dystonic contrac-

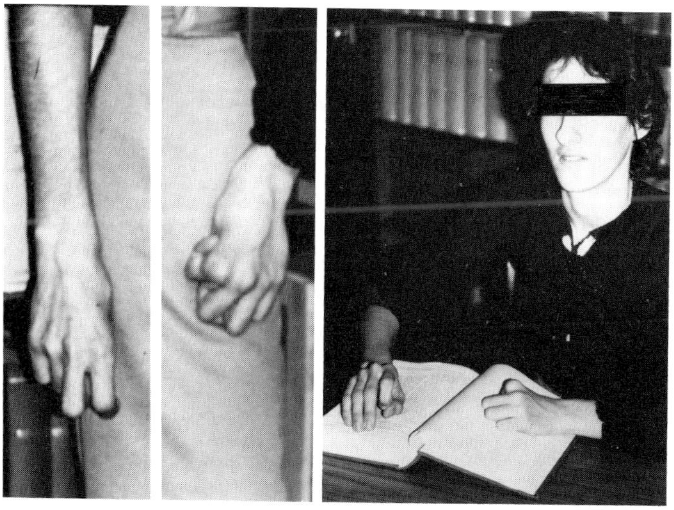

Figure 15–11. Contractures of the fingers of patient M5 requiring surgical correction.

tures of the feet or hands. In D4 and M6, lengthening of the Achilles tendon was necessary to correct equinovarus deformity that made walking all but impossible. In M5 (Fig. 15–11) the patient insisted on having her left hand operated on when penicillamine therapy had dramatically improved her almost total inability to walk, talk and eat. The surgeon, after sectioning the flexor profundus tendons as proximally as possible, and the flexor superficialis tendons as distally as possible, sutured each superficialis to its profundus under the appropriate degree of tension and released the intrinsic muscles of the thumb and index fingers, which had been replaced with scar tissue in many areas.

6. *Periodontal and reconstructive dental treatment.* These types of treatment are commonly required, perhaps because the teeth and supporting structures suffer the effects of dystonic jaw muscles, a mouth often held open, and poor oral hygiene due in part to patients' physical disabilities.[121]

REFERENCES

1. Walshe, J. M.: Wilson's disease. New oral therapy. Lancet *I*:25–26, 1956.
2. Sternlieb, I., and Scheinberg, I. H.: Penicillamine therapy in hepatolenticular degeneration. JAMA *189*:748–754, 1964.
3. Goldstein, N. P., and Gross, J. B.: Treatment of Wilson's disease. *In* Clinical Neuropharmacology. Ed. by H. L. Klawans, Raven Press, New York, pp. 99–112, 1977.
4. Boudin, G., Pépin, B., and Barraine, R.: Notre expérience du traitement de la maladie de Wilson par la pénicillamine. Bull. Soc. Méd. Hôp. Paris *114*:631–642, 1963.
5. Strickland, G. T., Blackwell, R. Q., and Watten, R. H.: Metabolic studies in Wilson's disease. Evaluation of efficacy of chelation therapy in respect to copper balance. Amer. J. Med. *51*:31–40, 1971.
6. Sass-Kortsak, A.: Wilson's disease: A treatable liver disease in children. Pediat. Clin. N. Amer. *22*:963–984, 1975.
7. Lange, J.: Zur Diagnostik und Therapie der hepatozerebralen Degeneration (Morbus Wilson). Dtsch. Med. Wschr. *88*:896–900, 1963.

8. Deiss, A., Lynch, R. E., Lee, G. R., and Cartwright, G. E.: Long-term therapy of Wilson's disease. Ann. Intern. Med. *75*:57–65, 1971.
9. Walshe, J. M.: Copper chelation in patients with Wilson's disease. A comparison of penicillamine and triethylene tetramine dihydrochloride. Quart J. Med. *42*:441–452, 1973.
9a. Hartl, J. and Hauftová, D.: Results of long-term therapy of Wilson's disease. Čs. Neurol. Neurochir. *45*:117–123, 1982.
10. Bergstrom, R. F., Kay, D. R., Harkcom, T. M., and Wagner, J. G.: Penicillamine kinetics in normal subjects. Clin. Pharmacol. Therapeut. *30*:404–413, 1981.
11. Gibbs, K., and Walshe, J. M.: Penicillamine and pyridoxine requirements in man. Lancet *I*:175–179, 1966.
12. Jaffe, I., Altman, K., and Merryman, P.: The antipyridoxine effect of penicillamine in man. J. Clin. Invest. *43*:1869–1873, 1964.
13. Hook, L., and Brandt, I. K.: Copper content of some low-copper foods. J. Amer. Dietet. Assoc. *49*:202–203, 1966.
14. Lawler, M. R., and Jelenc, M. A.: Recipes for low-copper diets. J. Amer. Dietet. Assoc. *57*:420–422, 1970.
15. Committee on Medical and Biological Effects of Environmental Pollutants: Human copper metabolism. *In* Copper. National Academy of Sciences, Washington, D.C., 1977, pp. 29–54.
16. Sussman, W., and Scheinberg, I. H.: Disappearance of Kayser-Fleischer rings. Arch. Ophthalmol. *82*:738–741, 1969.
17. Walshe, J. M.: The eye in Wilson's disease. *In* Birth Defects, Original Article Series, Vol. XII, No. 3. Ed. by Bergsma, D., Scheinberg, I. H., and Sternlieb, I. The National Foundation—March of Dimes, New York, 1976, pp. 187–189.
18. Wiebers, D. O., Hollenhorst, R. W., and Goldstein, N. P.: The ophthalmologic manifestations of Wilson's disease. Mayo Clin. Proc. *52*:409–416, 1977.
19. Schoenberger, M., and Ellis, P. P.: Disappearance of Kayser-Fleischer rings after liver transplantation. Arch. Ophthalmol. *97*:1914–1915, 1979.
20. Sternlieb, I.: Present status of diagnosis and prophylaxis of asymptomatic patients with Wilson's disease. *In* Diseases of the Liver and Biliary Tract. Ed. by Leevy, C. M. S. Karger, Basel, 1976, pp. 137–142.
21. Berry, W. R., Aronson, A. E., Darley, F. L., and Goldstein, N. P.: Effect of penicllamine therapy and low-copper diet on dysarthria in Wilson's disease (hepatolenticular degeneration). Mayo Clin. Proc. *49*:405–408, 1974.
21a. Sternlieb, I., Scheinberg, I. H., and Walshe, J. M.: Bleeding oesophageal varices in patients with Wilson's disease. Lancet *I*:638–641, 1970.
21b. Mareček, Z., Heyrovsky, A., and Volek, V.: The effect of long term treatment with penicillamine on the copper content in the liver in patients with Wilson's disease. Acta Hepato-Gastroenterol. *22*:292–296, 1975.
22. Grand, R. J., and Vawter, G. F.: Juvenile Wilson's disease: Histologic and functional studies during penicillamine therapy. J. Pediatr. *87*:1161–1170, 1975.
23. Sternlieb, I., and Feldmann, G.: Effects of anticopper therapy on hepatolenticular mitochondria in patients with Wilson's disease. Gastroenterology *71*:457–461, 1976.
24. Falkmer, S., Samuelson, G., and Sjölin, S.: Penicillamine-induced normalization of clinical signs and liver morphology and histochemistry in a case of Wilson's disease. Pediatrics *45*:260–268, 1970.
25. Scheinberg, I. H.: Human health effects of copper. *In* Copper in the Environment. Ed. by Nriagu, J. O. J. Wiley & Sons, New York, 1979, pp. 17–31.
26. Scheinberg, I. H., and Sternlieb, I.: Pregnancy in penicillamine treated patients with Wilson's disease. N. Engl. J. Med. *293*:1300–1302, 1975.
27. Walshe, J. M.: Wilson's disease (hepatolenticular degeneration). *In* Handbook of Clinical Neurology. Metabolic and Deficiency Diseases of the Nervous System, Vol. 27, Part I. Ed. by Vinken, P. J., Bruyn, G. W., and Klawans, H. L. American Elsevier Publishing Co., New York, 1976, pp. 379–414.
28. Deiss, A., Lee, G. R., and Cartwright, G. E.: Hemolytic anemia in Wilson's disease. Ann. Intern. Med. *73*:413–418, 1970.
29. Barbeau, A., and Friesen, H.: Treatment of Wilson's disease with L-DOPA after failure with penicillamine. Lancet *I*:1180–1181, 1970.
30. Gelmers, H. J., Troost, J., and Willemse, J.: Wilson's disease: Modification by L-DOPA. Neuropaediatrie *4*:453–457, 1973.
31. Berio, A.: Favourable results from the association of L-DOPA, amantadine and penicillamine in a child with Wilson's disease. I.R.C.S. *2*:1326, 1974.
32. Morgan, J. P., Preziosi, T. J., and Bianchine, J. R.: Ineffectiveness of L-DOPA as a supplement to penicillamine in a case of Wilson's disease. Lancet *II*:659, 1970.
33. Storch, W., Lössner, J., and Ruchholtz, U.: Schwerwiegende Nebenwirkungen unter D-Penicillamintherapie der Wilsonschen Erkankung. Psychiat. Neurol. Med. Psychol. (Leipzig) *31*:531–538, 1979.
34. Walshe, J. M.: Wilson's disease review. *In* Biochemistry of Copper. Ed. by Peisach, J., Aisen, P., and Blumberg, W. Academic Press, New York, 1966, pp. 475–498.
35. Strickland, G. T.: Febrile penicillamine eruption. Arch. Neurol. *26*:474, 1972.
36. Mirouze, J., Jaffiol, C., and Mary, P.: Etude clinique thérapeutique et isotopique d'une maladie de Wilson familiale. Désensibilisation à la d-pénicillamine. Marseille Méd. *106*:495–503, 1969.

37. Lössner, J., Eichner, B., Bachmann, H., Biesold, D., and Günther, K.: Verlaufsbeobachtung und Rehabiltation im klinischen Stadium der Wilsonschen Erkrankung. Psychiat. Neurol. Med. Psychol. (Leipzig) *26*:661–675, 1974.
38. Crawhall, J. C.: Proteinuria in d-penicillamine-treated rheumatoid arthritis. J. Rheumatol. *8*:(Suppl. 7):161–163, 1981.
39. Elsas, L. J., Hayslett, J. P., Spargo, B. H., Durant, J. L., and Rosenberg, L. E.: Wilson's disease with reversible renal tubular dysfunction. Correlation with proximal tubular ultrastructure. Ann. Intern. Med. *75*:427–433, 1971.
40. Lössner, J., Storch, W., Bachmann, H., Biesold, D., and Kuhn, H. J.: Untersuchungen zur Wilsonschen Erkankung in der DDR. III. Diagnose und Therapie. Zschr. f. Ges. Inn. Med. *35*:161–166, 1980.
41. Bacon, P. A., Tribe, C. R., Mackenzie, J. C., Verrier Jones, J., Cummings, R. H., and Amer, B.: Penicillamine nephropathy in rheumatoid arthritis. Quart. J. Med. *45*:661–684, 1976.
42. Sternlieb, I.: Penicillamine and the nephrotic syndrome. Results in patients with hepatolenticular degeneration. JAMA *198*:1311–1312, 1966.
43. Boudin, G., and Pépin, B.: Les accidents possibles de la pénicillamine au cours du traitement de la maladie de Wilson. Bull. Acad. Nat. Méd. (Paris) *156*:375–379, 1972.
44. Dubois, R. S., Rodgerson, D. O., Slovis, T. L., Hambidge, K. M., and Bianchi, T. A.: Triethylene tetramine dihydrochloride in Wilson's disease. Lancet *II*:775, 1970.
45. Harders, H., and Cohnen, E.: Preparation of and clinical experiences with trien for treatment of Wilson's disease in absolute intolerance of D-penicillamine. Proc. Roy. Soc. Med. *70*:(Suppl. 3):10–18, 1977.
46. Boudin, G., Pépin, B., Godeau, P., Vernant, J.-C., and Gouerou, H.: Lupus erythémateux induit par la pénicillamine au cours d'une maladie de Wilson. Ann. Méd. Interne. (Paris) *122*:269–273, 1971.
47. Caille, B., Harpey, J.-P., Lejeune, C., Sudre, Y., and Turpin, R.: Syndrome lupique induit par D-pénicillamine au cours d'une maladie de Wilson. Etude clinique d'une observation. Ann. Méd. Interne (Paris) *122*:255–260, 1971.
48. Walshe, J. M.: Penicillamine and the SLE syndrome. J. Rheumatol. *8*(Suppl. 7):155–160, 1981.
49. Heinrich, F., and Kaltenbach, M.: Morbus Wilson unter dem Bild einer Panhämozytopenie. Med. Klin. *60*:499–502, 1965.
50. Ahmed, F., Sumalop, V., Spain, D. M., and Tobin, M. S.: Thrombohemolytic, thrombocytopenic purpura during penicillamine therapy. Arch. Intern. Med. *132*:1292–1293, 1978.
51. Gollan, J. L., Hussein, S., Hoffbrand, A. V., and Sherlock, S.: Red cell aplasia following prolonged D-penicillamine therapy. J. Clin. Pathol. *29*:135–139, 1976.
52. Tu, J., Blackwell, R. Q., and Lee, P. F.: DL-penicillamine as a cause of optic axial neuritis. JAMA *185*:83–86, 1963.
53. Goldstein, N. P., Hollenhorst, R. W., Randall, P. V., and Gross, J. B.: Possible relationship of optic neuritis, Wilson's disease and DL-penicillamine therapy. JAMA *196*:734–735, 1966.
54. Damaske, E., and Althoff, W.: Neuritis optici bei einem Kind mit Wilsonscher Krankheit. Klin. Mbl. Augenheilk. *160*:168–175, 1972.
55. Sternlieb, I., Bennett, B., and Scheinberg, I. H.: D-penicillamine induced Goodpasture's syndrome in Wilson's disease. Ann. Intern. Med. *82*:673–675, 1975.
56. Sternlieb, I., Fisher, M., and Scheinberg, I. H.: Penicillamine-induced skin lesions. J. Rheumatol. *8*(Suppl. 7):149–154, 1981.
57. Katz, R.: Penicillamine induced skin lesions. A possible example of human lathyrism. Arch. Dermatol. *95*:196–198, 1967.
58. Kueppers, F., and Daniels, F., Jr.: Penicillamine-induced skin lesions in patients with Wilson's disease. Cutis *5*:35–39, 1969.
59. Nimni, M. E.: Mechanism of inhibition of collagen cross-linking by penicillamine. Proc. Roy. Soc. Med. *70*(Suppl. 3):65–72, 1977.
60. Morris, J. J., Seifter, E., Rettura, G., Geever, E. F., and Levenson, S. M.: Effect of penicillamine upon wound healing. J. Surg. Res. *9*:143–149, 1969.
61. Charlebois, G., Cadotte, M., and Barbeau, A.: Cutis hyperelastica après administration prolongée de pénicillamine chez une patiente atteinte de la maladie de Wilson. Union Méd. Can. *101*:839–895, 1972.
62. Pass, F., Goldfischer, S., Sternlieb, I., and Scheinberg, I. H.: Elastosis perforans serpiginosa after penicillamine therapy for Wilson's disease. Arch. Dermatol. *108*:713–715, 1973.
63. Kirsch, N., and Hukill, P. B.: Elastosis perforans serpiginosa by penicillamine. Electron microscopic observations. Arch. Dermatol. *113*:630–635, 1977.
64. Bardach, H., Gebhart, W., Niebauer, G.: "Lumpy-bumpy" elastic fibers in the skin and lungs of a patient with penicillamine-induced elastosis perforans serpiginosa. J. Cut. Pathol. *6*:243–252, 1979.
64a. Rosenblum, G. A.: Liquid nitrogen cryotherapy in a case of elastosis perforans serpiginosa. J. Amer. Acad. Dermatol. *8*:718–721, 1983.
65. Degros, R., Touraine, R., Belaich, S., and Revuz, J.: Pemphigus chez un malade traité par pénicillamine pour maladie de Wilson. Bull. Soc. Franç. Dermatol. *76*:751–753, 1969.
66. Eisenberg, E., Ballow, M., Wolfe, S. H., Krutchkoff, D. L., and Tanzer, J. M.: Pemphigus-like mucosal lesions: A side effect of penicillamine therapy. Oral Surg. Oral Med. Oral Pathol. *51*:409–414, 1981.

67. Van de Staak, W. J. B. M., Cotton, D. W. K., Jonckheer-Venneste, M. M. H., and Boerbooms, A. M. T. H.: Lichenoid eruption following penicillamine. Dermatologia *150*:372–374, 1975.
68. Bennett, R. A., and Harbilas, E.: Wilson's disease with aseptic meningitis and penicillamine-related cheilosis. Arch. Intern. Med. *120*:374–376, 1967.
69. Masters, C. L., Dawkins, R. L., Zilko, P. J., Simpson, J. A., Leedman, R. J., and Lindstrom, J.: Penicillamine-associated myasthenia gravis, antiacetylcholine receptor and antistriational antibodies. Amer. J. Med. *63*:689–694, 1977.
70. Czlonkowska, A.: Myasthenia syndrome during penicillamine treatment. Brit. Med. J. *2*:726–727, 1975.
71. Henkin, R. I., Keiser, H. R., Jaffe, I. A., Sternlieb, I., and Scheinberg, I. H.: Decreased taste sensitivity after D-penicillamine reversed by copper administration. Lancet *II*:1268–1271, 1967.
72. Henkin, R. I., and Bradley, D. F.: Hypogeusiaa corrected by Ni^{++} and Zn^{++}. Life Sci. *9*:701–709, 1970.
73. Proesman, W., Jaeken, J., and Eckels, R.: D-penicillamine induced IgA deficiency in Wilson's disease. Lancet *II*:804–805, 1976.
74. Hjalmarson, O., Hanson, L. A., and Nilsson, L.-A.: IgA deficiency during penicillamine treatment. Brit. Med. J. *I*:549, 1977.
75. Forrest, R. D., Bostrom, H., and Dahlberg, P. A.: IgA deficiency during penicillamine treatment. Brit. Med. J. *I*:777, 1977.
76. Michel, F.-B., Bousquet, J., Robinet-Levy, M., and Mary, P.: Déficit immunitaire lors d'un traitement par D-pénicillamine. Nouv. Presse Méd. *6*:3546–4537, 1977.
77. Strickland, G. T., and Leu, M. L.: Wilson's disease. Clinical and laboratory manifestations in 40 patients. Medicine *54*:113–137, 1975.
77a. Czlonkowska, A.: The effect of long-term treatment with D-penicillamine on the humoral immune response in patients with Wilson's disease. Mat. Med. Polona *1*:1–3, 1976.
77b. Gilman, P. A., and Holtzman, N. A.: Acute lymphoblastic leukemia in a patient receiving penicillamine for Wilson's disease. JAMA *248*:467–468, 1982.
78. Klepach, G. L., and Wray, S. H.: Bilateral serous retinal detachment with thrombocytopenia during penicillamine therapy. Ann. Ophthalmol. *13*:201–203, 1981.
79. Dingle, J., and Havener, W. H.: Ophthalmoscopic changes in a patient with Wilson's disease during long-term penicillamine therapy. Ann. Ophthalmol. *10*:1227–1230, 1978.
80. Hamlyn, A. M., Gollan, J. L., Douglas, A. P., and Sherlock, S.: Fulminant Wilson's disease with haemolysis and renal failure: copper studies and assessment of dialysis regimens. Brit. Med. J. *II*:660–663, 1977.
80a. Guerin, J. M., Raux, M., Meresse, S., and Lamotte, M.: Epuration du cuivre par dialyse péritoneale dans la maladie de Wilson. Sem. Hôp. Paris *58*:613–615, 1982.
80b. Danks, D. M.: Penicillamine in Wilson's disease. Lancet *II*:435–436, 1982.
80c. Regan, P. A.: The nursing care of a patient with Wilson's disease. J. Neurosurg. *3*:15–25, 1971.
81. Denny-Brown, D., and Porter, H.: The effect of BAL (2,3-dimercaptopropanol) on hepatolenticular degeneration (Wilson's disease). N. Engl. J. Med. *245*:917–925, 1951.
82. Cumings, J. N.: Effects of B.A.L. in hepatolenticular degeneration. Brain *74*:10–22, 1951.
83. Sternlieb, I., and Scheinberg, I. H.: The prevention of Wilson's disease in asymptomatic patients. N. Engl. J. Med. *278*:352–359, 1968.
84. Lange, J.: Über den klinisch asymptomatischen Morbus Wilson. Dtsch. Med. Wschr. *87*:541–544, 1962.
85. Levi, A. J., Sherlock, S., Scheuer, P. J., and Cumings, J. N.: Presymptomatic Wilson's disease. Lancet *II*:575–579, 1967.
86. Tu, J.-B., Cooper, W. C., Blackwell, R. Q., and Hou, T.-Y.: Treatment of hepatolenticular degeneration (Wilson's disease) in the asymptomatic stage. Neurology *15*:402–408, 1965.
87. Jérôme, H., and Sternlieb, I.: La détection préclinique de la maladie de Wilson. Arch. Franç. Pédiat. *23*:669–677, 1966.
88. Bocquet, L., Jérôme, H., and Turpin, R.: Les lésions hépatiques de la maladie de Wilson préclinique. Intérêt du dépistage. Sem. Hôp. Paris *43*:1369–1374, 1967.
89. Wewalka, F.: Morbus Wilson. Einführung in die aktuellen Probleme (Frühdiagnose und Therapie). Wiener Zschr. Inn. Med. *12*:461–466, 1967.
90. Arima, M., Komiya, K., Fujusawa, A., and Matsuoka, K.: Prevention of Wilson's disease in asymptomatic patients. Proc. Austral. Assoc. Neurol. *5*:197–201, 1968.
91. Kittoe, K., and Colombo, J. P.: Präsymptomatische und hepatische Form des Morbus Wilson im Kindesalter. Langzeitbehandlung mit D-Penicillamin. Praxis *57*:1–22, 1968.
92. Arima, M., and Komiya, K.: Prevention of Wilson's disease: a long-term follow-up. Paediat. Univ. Tokyo *18*:22–24, 1970.
93. Campanella, G., Gillardi, U., and Germinario, L.: Contributi allo studio della degenerazione epatolenticolare (Morbo di Wilson). I. Despistage e diagnosi precoce. Acta Neurol. (Naples) *26*:403–422, 1971.
94. Kuncova, Z., Dittrich, J., Nevsimalova, S., Mareček, Z., and Heyrovsky, A.: Diagnostika asymptomatickych forem hepatolentikularni degenerace. Cesk. Pediat. *26*:166–169, 1971.
95. Lössner, J., Bachmann, H., Eichner, B., Biesold, D., and Günther, K.: Diagnostische und therapeutische Aspekte der Wilsonschen Erkrankung in praeklinischen Stadium. Psychiatr. Neurol. Med. Psychol. *25*:266–275, 1973.
96. Schmid-Rüter, E., Feist, D., Wesch, H., Rossner, J. A., and Schärer, K.: Präsymptomatischer

Morbus Wilson. Diagnose, Behandlung und Familienuntersuchung. Dtsch. Med. Wschr. *98*:1698–1703, 1973.

97. Hamza, B., and El Kamel, M.: A propros de deux cas de maladie de Wilson dépistés au stade infraclinique. Traitement précoce et prolongé à la pénicillamine. Résultat. Tunis Méd. *52*:29–31, 1974.
98. Tiwary, C. M., Rennert, O. M., and Garnica, A.: Penicillamine in prevention of symptomatic Wilson's disease: 8 year follow-up in two sibs. Indian Pediat. *12*:189–195, 1975.
99. Streifler, M., and Feldman, S.: Effect of dimercaprol (BAL) in hepatolenticular degeneration: Report of a case with clinical electroencephalographic study. Arch. Neurol. Psychiat. *69*:84–90, 1953.
100. Walshe, J. M.: Treatment of Wilson's disease with trientine (triethylene tetramine) dihydrochloride. Lancet *I*:643–647, 1982.
100a. Hayes, A. H., Jr.: Triethylene dihydrochloride for treatment of penicillamine-intolerant patients with Wilson's disease; Invitation to submit new drug application. Fed. Reg. *47*(186):42175–42176, 1982.
101. Walshe, J. M.: An assessment of the treatment of Wilson's disease with triethylene tetramine 2 HCl (Trien 2 HCl). *In* Biological Aspects of Metal Related Diseases. Ed. by Sarkar, B. Raven Press, New York, 1982.
102. Sass-Kortsak, A.: Treatment of Wilson's disease with triethylene tetramine dihydrochloride. A case report. Dev. Pharmacol. Ther. *1*:318–324, 1980.
103. Hoogenraad, T. U., Koevoet, R., and de Ruyter Korver, E. G. W. M.: Oral zinc sulphate as long-term treatment in Wilson's disease (Hepatolenticular degeneration). Eur. Neurol. *18*:205–211, 1979.
104. Hoogeneraad, T. U., van den Hamer, C. J. A., Koevoet, R., and de Ruyter Korver, E. G. W. M.: Oral zinc in Wilson's disease. Lancet *II*:1262, 1978.
104a. Brewer, C. J., Prasad, A. S., Cossack, Z. T., and Rabbani, P. I.: Treatment of Wilson's disease with oral zinc. Clin. Res. *29*:758a, 1981.
104b. Walshe, J. M.: Personal communication, 1982.
105. Sunderman, F. W., Jr., White, J. C., and Sunderman, F. W.: Metabolic balance studies in hepatolenticular degeneration treated with diethylcarbamate. Amer. J. Med. *34*:875–888, 1963.
106. Hsia, Y. E., Combs, J. T., Hook, L., and Brandt, I. K.: Hepatolenticular degeneration: the comparative effectiveness of D-penicillamine, potassium sulfide, and diethylthiocarbamate as decoppering agents. J. Pediat. *68*:921–926, 1966.
107. Lang, H. D., Reichenmiller, H. E., Tigges, F.-J., Braun, H. J., and Golisch, G.: EEG-Veränderungen unter Natriumdiäthyldithiocarbamat-Behandlung bei zwei Fällen von Morbus Wilson. Med. Klin. *67*:916–921, 1972.
108. Boudin, G., and Pépin, B.: Essai de traitement de la maladie de Wilson par le diéthyl-dithiocarbamate de sodium. Bull. Soc. Méd. Hôp. (Paris) *116*:843–845, 1965.
109. Konovalov, N. V., Mittelstedt, A. A., Bauman, L. K., and Gotovtzeva, E. V.: The metabolism of copper in hepatolenticular degeneration and treatment with thiols. Zh. Nevropatol. Psikhiatr. (Moscow) *57*:39–48, 1957.
110. Konovalov, N. V., and Gotovtzeva, E. V.: Treatment of hepatolenticular degeneration. Zh. Nevropatol. Psikhiatr. (Moscow) *58*:897–906, 1958.
111. Melnichuk, P. V., Choclov, A. P., and Roshchina, N. A.: On the use of metal antagonists for the correction of copper metabolism in patients with hepatocerebral dystrophy. Zh. Nevropatol. Psikhiatr. (Moscow) *80*:372–376, 1980.
112. Sunderman, F. W., Hohnadel, D. C., Evenson, M. A., Wannamaker, B. B., and Dahl, D. S.: Excretion of copper in sweat of patients with Wilson's disease during sauna bathing. Ann. Clin. Lab. Sci. *4*:407–412, 1974.
113. Cooper, I. S.: Cryogenic surgery of the basal ganglia. JAMA *181*:600–604, 1962.
114. Mingrino, S., and Pavan, L.: Possibilità di trattamento della malattia di Wilson con talamolisi stereotassica. Giorn. Psich. Neuropatol. *46*:487–493, 1968.
115. Mundinger, F.: Phaenomenologie der wichtigsten pyramidal extrapyramidal motorischen Syndrome. Operations-Indikation und Resultate. II. Z. Allgemein. Med. *50*:838–845, 1974.
116. Spissu, A., Giagheddu, M., and Masala, C.: Impiego della chirurgia stereotassica nel trattamento della degenerazione epato-lenticulare. Riv. Neurol. *47*:465–472, 1977.
117. Bondarchuk, A. N., Borodkin, Y. S., Vakharlovsky, V. G., Neifakh, S. A., and Smirnov, V. M.: Complex medicamentous treatment of hepatolenticular degeneration. Vopr. Neirokhir. (Moscow) *1*:40–44, 1975.
118. Bennek, J., and Keller, E.: Morbus Wilson: Erfolgreiche Aszitesbehandlung durch einen LeVeen-Shunt (ein kasuistischer Beitrag). Z. Kinderchir. *29*:164–170, 1980.
119. Starzl, T. E., Iwatsuki, S., Van Thiel, D. H., Gartner, J. C., Zitelli, B. J., Malatack, J. J., Schade, R. R., Shaw, B. W., Jr., Hakala, T. R., Rosenthal, J. T., and Porter, K. A.: Evolution of liver transplantation. Hepatology *2*:614–636, 1982.
120. Dubois, R. S., Giles, G., Rodgerson, D. O., Lilly, J., Martineau, G., Halgrimson, C. G., Schroter, G., Starzl, T. E., Sternlieb, I., and Scheinberg, I. H.: Orthotopic liver transplantation for Wilson's disease. Lancet *I*:505–508, 1971.
120a. Sternlieb, I.: Wilson's disease: Indications for transplants. Hepatology, 1983 (in press).
121. Mestrom, T. J. H., and Spanauf, A. J.: The dental management of a partially edentulous patient suffering from hepatolenticular degeneration (Wilson's disease). Austr. Dent. J. *26*:153–155, 1981.

CHAPTER 16

ARE THERE RISKS TO PARENTHOOD IN WILSON'S DISEASE?

When it became clear, by the mid-1960s, that it was possible to restore the majority of patients with Wilson's disease to normal health, patients and their physicians began to assess the risks that might be associated with parenthood. Effective therapy, which also ended the multiple miscarriages that are frequently an accompaniment of untreated Wilson's disease,[1-3] compelled facing the issue. Early fears that patients, by reproducing, might increase significantly the incidence of the WD gene in the human gene pool or transmit the disease to their children could be shown to be almost baseless once the autosomal recessive character of the WD gene and the rarity of its incidence were known. The worldwide prevalence of heterozygous carriers of one WD gene is about 1 in 90, whereas the incidence of patients—abnormal homozygotes—is about 1 in 30,000 (see Chapter 2). Assuming equal reproductive rates of patients and carriers, there will be one heterozygote born to a patient for every 167 heterozygotes born to carriers.

Nor is the likelihood great that Wilson's disease will develop in the child of a patient. The a priori probability that each successful pregnancy resulting from the nonconsanguineous mating of a patient will terminate in the birth of an abnormally homozygous infant—another patient—is about 1 in 180. Over the past 30 years we have seen two instances of this in approximately 500 patients with Wilson's disease (T1, Table 16–1; and T3, Table 16–2). Of course, if a parent is known to have Wilson's disease, it is mandatory that the diagnosis be confirmed or ruled out in the infant soon after the first year of life, so that an affected child can be treated while asymptomatic.

The two risks that were much more troublesome were that pregnancy might worsen a woman's Wilson's disease, or that its treatment with penicillamine might affect her child. When we were asked about these risks by a patient in 1974 there already was evidence of the danger of the first in the literature[4,5] and in another patient of ours, M2, for whom abortion had proven necessary because of life-threatening esophageal variceal hemorrhage.

As for the second risk, penicillamine treatment of a pregnant woman with cystinuria had been reported to have caused a connective tissue defect in her child.[6] Although it was possible that this might have been coincidental,[7] reasonable concern persisted about the possibilities that penicillamine might adversely affect fetal connective tissue, induce fetal copper deficiency or result in teratogenesis. (Coincidental occurrence of the latter is also possible. For example, one woman—before the diagnosis and treatment of her Wilson's disease—delivered a baby girl with "a transverse reduction limb defect (hemimelia) of her left upper limb."[7a]) Indeed, although not previously remarked upon to our knowledge, it was even conceivable that long-term treatment of men with Wilson's disease could affect spermatogenesis, with teratogenic effects in their children.

From the literature, supplemented by correspondence with physicians,[1,2,5,8–17] and from previously unreported observations made in 20 female and 14 male patients of ours who have become parents (Tables 16–1 and 16–2), we have analyzed the courses and outcomes of 104 pregnancies carried to term in 69 women with Wilson's disease, and of 34 successful pregnancies fathered by 14 patients.

EFFECTS OF PREGNANCY ON THE MOTHER

Seven complications of these 104 pregnancies were almost certainly unrelated to the patients' Wilson's disease,[1,2,9] but the courses of five pregnancies are relevant.

1. During the second pregnancy of K1 (Table 16–1) the hemoglobin dropped to 8 g/dl with simultaneous elevations of her reticulocyte count to 3.7 per cent and serum bilirubin to 4.4 mg/dl immediately after delivery of a normal 7 lb 15 oz girl. Penicillamine had been continued throughout pregnancy but at only 0.5 g/day. Recovery was swift as the dose of penicillamine was raised to 1.0 g/day.

2. Severe hemolytic anemia occurred in the fifth month of pregnancy in a woman, D7, whose penicillamine was discontinued before she became pregnant. Reinstitution of penicillamine therapy was accompanied by cessation of the hemolysis.[5]

These two episodes of hemolytic anemia were probably due to reduction or withdrawal of penicillamine dosage, since maternal hemolytic anemia is an unusual complication of pregnancy but is not uncommon in inadequately treated Wilson's disease.

3. There was exacerbation of the liver disease of one woman whose Wilson's disease had produced advanced portal hypertension and in whom penicillamine treatment was discontinued before she became pregnant.[12]

4. In one patient, in whom penicillamine treatment was discontinued at the end of the first trimester, hepatic decompensation developed and progressed despite reinstitution of penicillamine following delivery of a normal boy. She died two years later.

TABLE 16–1. Effects of Penicillamine Treatment on the Course and Outcome of Pregnancies in Women with Wilson's Disease (Authors' Patients)

Case	Prior Penicillamine (g/day)	Pencillamine in Pregnancy (g/day)	Infant at Birth	Comment
D1	1.0	1.0	Normal girl	
D1	1.0	1.0 to 7th mo.	Normal girl	
D1	None for 3 yr.	0.5 to 4th mo.	Normal boy	
J2	1.0	1.0	Normal boy	
J2	1.0	0.75	Normal boy	
J2	1.0	0.75	Normal boy	
K1	0.5–1.0	0.5	Normal boy	
K1	0.5–0.75	0.5	Normal girl	Maternal hemolysis at term
S2	0–1.0, erratic	0.75	Normal boy	3 days of toxemia in hospital
S2	0–1.0, erratic	Little, if any	Normal girl	
S3	No	No	Normal boy	
S3	1.0	1.0	Normal girl	
P2	1.0	1.0	Normal girl	
L1	0.75	0.75	Normal boy	
H1*	0.75	0.75	Normal girl	
D2	No	No	Normal infant	
D2	No	No	Normal infant	

O1	No	No	Normal boy
O1	No	No	Normal boy
H2	No	No	Normal boy
T1	No	No	Normal girl, but asymptomatic WD diagnosed at age 12 (Case T2)
C1	No	No	Normal girl
A2	No	No	Normal girl
E1	No	No	Normal girl
E1	No	No	Normal girl
E2	No	No	Normal girl
L2	No	No	Normal boy
L2	No	No	Normal boy
M3	No	No	Normal girl
M3	No	No	Normal boy
P3	No	No	Normal girl
M4	No	No	2 normal children
Total infants delivered:			33

*Pregnancy followed treatment with clomiphene citrate.

TABLE 16–2. Absence of Adverse Effects on Infants Fathered by Penicillamine-treated or Untreated Patients with Wilson's Disease (Authors' Patients)

	Treatment Before Pregnancy		
Case	*Duration (years)*	*Penicillamine (g/day)*	Infant
S4	10	1.0; then al-	Normal boy
S4	11	most zero from	Normal boy
S4	12	16 to 20 yr.	Normal boy
S5	12	1.0	Normal boy
S5	13	1.0	Normal boy
S5	14	1.0	Normal boy
L3		None	Normal girl
L3		None	Normal girl
L3	6	1.0	Normal girl
S1		None	Normal boy
S1		None	Normal girl
S1	4	1.0	Normal girl
K2	10	2.0–3.0; and	Normal boy
K2	12	1.0 after 10 yr.	Normal boy
R1	8	1.0; erratic	Normal girl
A3	>10	0.75–2.0	Normal boy
A3	>10	0.75–2.0	Normal girl
F1	>10	1.0	Normal boy
F1	>10	1.0	Normal boy
F1	>10	1.0	Normal boy
F2	>10	1.0–2.0	Normal boy
F2	>10	1.0–2.0	Normal boy
T3		None	Normal girl, but WD diagnosed at age 10 (case D1)
Y1		None	Normal (5 children)
D3		None	Normal girl
P4		None	Normal (3 children)
G1		None	Normal boys (2)
Total infants fathered:			34

The worsening of liver disease in these two patients may have been partly caused by their limited functional hepatic reserve, as well as by the withdrawal of penicillamine. Unrelated to pregnancy are other instances we have seen in which such hepatic decompensation was irreversible despite reinstitution of penicillamine treatment.

5. Miscarriage was threatened at the tenth week of pregnancy in a woman in whom penicillamine treatment was discontinued four weeks previously. Reinstitution of the drug at the twelfth week was followed by mild pre-eclampsia at term and delivery of a normal girl.[2]

OUTCOMES OF 104 PREGNANCIES IN WOMEN WITH WILSON'S DISEASE

Only two of the neonates exhibited an abnormality.

One infant, whose mother received 1.5 g/day of penicillamine, was observed to have cutis laxa; by two months after birth the infant's skin was normal.[15]

The male infant of a woman who received 0.5 g/day penicillamine throughout pregnancy was hypoxic at birth but, except for a "moderate pansystolic bruit, suggestive of a ventricular septal defect," was normal at nine weeks of age."[15]

OUTCOMES OF 34 PREGNANCIES FATHERED BY PATIENTS WITH WILSON'S DISEASE

All of these children were normal. The oldest is now more than 30 years old.

CONCLUSIONS

We believe, from these data, that there is no contraindication to pregnancy in a woman with Wilson's disease who has no significant hepatic dysfunction, provided adequate penicillamine therapy is continued throughout gestation. Although cirrhosis increases the risk of spontaneous abortion, prematurity and stillbirth,[18] these risks seem to be less in women with Wilson's disease. The frequent miscarriages seen in untreated women with Wilson's disease are less likely to be due to their cirrhosis than to free copper in intrauterine secretions, since miscarriages are unusual in penicillamine-treated patients with low concentrations of free serum copper.[1–3] As we learned from our case in which abortion was necessary, prominent esophageal varices should alert the physician to the possibility of bleeding during pregnancy due to increased blood volume and intra-abdominal pressure from the enlarging uterus.

Obviously, women with Wilson's disease *can* have normal pregnancies *without* penicillamine therapy, since 13 of our patients (Table 16–1) and nine reported in the literature[2, 12, 17] gave birth to 29 normal infants following such pregnancies. There were no complications in any of the 13 women in Table 16–1 or in the one patient in Walshe's series,[2] all of whom were asymptomatic and untreated before they conceived. But in any woman with Wilson's disease symptomatic enough to have led to its diagnosis and treatment with penicillamine before pregnancy, treatment at a dose of 0.75 to 1.0 g daily should be continued throughout pregnancy. Withdrawal of the drug in these patients, as illustrated by the five cases described above, is dangerous to the mother, whereas its continued administration, also as documented above, is without appreciable risk to the fetus. If caesarean section is contemplated, the daily dose of penicillamine should be reduced to no more than 0.75 g.

These conclusions do not necessarily apply (though the observations reported by Lyle suggest that they probably do[19]) to women who receive penicillamine for other disorders. However, teratogenesis, observed in rats receiving penicillamine or trientine during pregnancy, has been ascribed to copper deficiency.[20, 21] To our knowledge copper deficiency has never been reported in penicillamine-treated patients with Wilson's disease or in infants of Wilsonian mothers whose treatment was continued during pregnancy. But since penicillamine can induce copper deficiency in individuals without Wilson's disease, the physician will want to consider these factors in deciding whether to continue use of the drug during pregnancy in women with cystinuria or rheumatoid arthritis.[22]

The treatment of Wilson's disease with trientine before and during pregnancy has been carried out in four patients of Walshe who have had six apparently uneventful pregnancies with no miscarriages. There were no abnormalities noted in the infants, and Walshe could not demonstrate any teratogenicity in mice given this drug before and during pregnancy.[23]

REFERENCES

1. Scheinberg, I. H., and Sternlieb, I.: Pregnancy in penicillamine-treated patients with Wilson's disease. N. Engl. J. Med. *293*:1300–1302, 1975.
2. Walshe, J. M.: Pregnancy in Wilson's disease. Quart. J. Med. *46*:73–83, 1977.
3. Klee, J. G.: Undiagnosed Wilson's disease as cause of unexplained miscarriage. Lancet *II*:423, 1979.
4. Scheinberg, I. H., and Sternlieb, I.: The long-term management of hepatolenticular degeneration (Wilson's disease). Amer. J. Med. *29*:316–333, 1960.
5. Deiss, A., Lee, G. R., and Cartwright, G. E.: Hemolytic anemia in Wilson's disease. Ann. Int. Med. *73*:413–418, 1970.
6. Mjolnerod, I. K., Rasmussen, K., Dommerud, S. A., and Gjeruldsen, S. T.: Congenital connective tissue defect probably due to D-penicillamine treatment in pregnancy. Lancet *I*:673–676, 1971.
7. Laver, M., and Fairley, K. F.: D-penicillamine treatment in pregnancy. Lancet *I*:1019–1020, 1971.
7a. Pappas, S. C.: Personal communication.
8. Tsuzuki, E., Scaff, M., Roitman, I., Neme, B., and Canelas, H. M.: Degeneracao hepatolenticular e gravidez. Rev. Hosp. Clin. Fac. Med. (São Paulo) *31*:35–38, 1976.
9. Gollan, J. L., Hussein, S., Hoffbrand, A. V., and Sherlock, S.: Red cell aplasia following prolonged D-penicillamine therapy. J. Clin. Pathol. *29*:135–139, 1976.
10. Shrand, H.: Personal communication.
11. Lederbogen, K.: Ergebnisse einer zehnjährigen Behandlung eines Morbus Wilson mit Metalcaptase. Abstracts of 84th Meeting Nordwestdtsch Ges. Inn. Med. (Hamburg), 1975.
12. Mareček, Z., and Graf, M.: Pregnancy in penicillamine-treated patients with Wilson's disease. N. Engl. J. Med. *295*:841–842, 1976.
13. Toulouse, R., Poirier, P. Y., de Villartay, A., and Kerisit, J.: Maladie de Wilson et grossesse. J. Gynecol. Obstet. Biol. Repr. *3*:1057–1062, 1974.
14. Fukuda, K., Ishii, A., Matsue, Y., Funaki, K., Hoshiai, H., and Maeda, S.: Pregnancy and delivery in penicillamine treated patients with Wilson's disease. Tohoku J. Exp. Med. *123*:279–285, 1977.
15. Master, C. J., Dawkins, R. L., Zilko, P. J., Simpson, J. A., Leedman, R. J., and Lindstrom, J.: Penicillamine-associated myasthenia gravis, antiacetylcholine receptor and antistriational antibodies. Amer. J. Med. *63*:689–694, 1977.
16. Linares, A., Zarranz, J. J., Rodriguez-Alarcon, J., and Diaz-Perez, J. L.: Reversible cutis laxa due to maternal penicillamine treatment. Lancet *II*:43, 1979.
17. Chapoy, P., Devaux, J., Ferracci, J. P., Mallet, P., and Louchet, E.: Approche biochimique de la pathologie du cuivre chez l'enfant. Journées Paris. Péd. 1978.
18. Cheng, Y.: Pregnancy in liver cirrhosis and/or portal hypertension. Amer. J. Obstet. Gynecol. *128*:812, 1977.
19. Lyle, W. H.: Penicillamine in pregnancy. Lancet *I*:606–607, 1978.
20. Keen, C. L., Mark-Savage, P., Lonnerdal, B., and Hurley, L. S.: Low-tissue copper and teratogenesis in rats resulting from D-penicillamine. Fed. Proc. *40*:917, 1981.
21. Keen, C. L., Cohen, N. L., Lonnerdal, B., and Hurley, L. S.: Low-tissue copper and teratogenesis in trientine-treated rats. Lancet *I*:1127, 1982.
22. Solomon, L., Abrams, G., Dinner, M., and Berman, L.: Neonatal abnormalities associated with D-penicillamine treatment during pregnancy. N. Engl. J. Med. *296*:54–55, 1977.
23. Walshe, J. M.: Treatment of Wilson's disease with trientine (triethylene tetramine) dihydrochloride. Lancet *I*:643–647, 1982.

INDEX OF PATIENT REFERENCES

INDEX

Page numbers in *italics* indicate illustrations. Page numbers followed by t indicate tables.

NO POSTAGE
NECESSARY
IF MAILED
IN THE
UNITED STATES

BUSINESS REPLY CARD

FIRST CLASS PERMIT NO. 101 PHILADELPHIA, PA

POSTAGE WILL BE PAID BY ADDRESSEE

W.B. SAUNDERS COMPANY
West Washington Square
Philadelphia, PA 19105